Stories of Healing
A Family Doctor's Journal

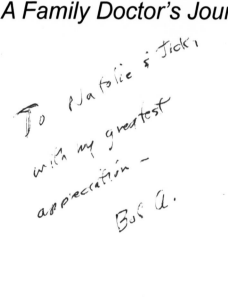

To Natalie & Jicki
with my greatest
appreciation —
Bob A.

Robert A. Anderson, MD

Stories of Healing
A Family Doctor's Journal

Cover and Interior Photographs by
Douglas R. Anderson, cinematographer
Edited by Joann M. Anderson

ISBN-13: 978-0-9837422-1-0

Anderson, Robert A.
Stories of Healing: *A Family Doctor's Journal*/Robert A. Anderson, MD

Library of Congress Control Number: 2011939883

First Edition October 2011

Printed in the United States of America

0 9 8 7 6 5 4 3 2 1

Starseed Publications
2204 E Grand Ave.
Everett, WA 98201

Dedication

I wish to extend my profound appreciation for my many patients who taught me much of what I know. The aid of my wife, Joann, has been invaluable in editing and proof-reading the text and bringing it to publication.

Legal Disclaimer

This book provides general information about medicine, health, and related topics. The information is offered for educational purposes only and represents vignettes of the author's experience in forty years of clinical medical practice. It does not offer explicit medical advice or instruction, and no health care decisions should be undertaken based solely on its contents. Readers should consult their own health care professionals on any matter regarding their own health and well being.

The views expressed in this book have no relation to those of any academic, hospital, clinical practice, or other institution with which the author is affiliated.

The author and publisher are not responsible for any injury resulting from the material presented herein. Health care practitioners should use appropriate judgment when making all clinical decisions.

Contents

Foreword

Bob Anderson, MD, has done more to advance integrative holistic medicine in America than almost anyone I know. He has been a modest and unsung hero of mine who has quietly contributed as much to the integrative holistic medicine movement as have more well-known leaders in the field such as Andrew Weil, Norm Shealy, Jim Gordon, and Larry Dossey.

Dr. Anderson has been the personal holistic physician to tens of thousands of patients; he has written four scholarly books documenting the science of holistic medicine; he has published extensively in journals; he has taught for many years at Bastyr University's Naturopathic Medicine program; he served as President of the American Holistic Medical Association; and he founded and served as the Executive Director of the American Board of Integrative Holistic Medicine.

Dr. Anderson has built on this lifetime of medical leadership and service with his latest publication, *Stories of Healing: A Family Doctor's Journal*. This powerful and poignant book describes the healing journeys of over forty of his patients. For those of us who love stories, this book is a gem. Each chapter is devoted to one patient's story of how healing emerged from that person's own body, mind, emotions, and spirit. Dr. Anderson discovered during his years of working with patients that his primary job was to enhance their self-healing capacity through compassion, good listening, and open-heartedness as he encouraged them to find meaning in their illness.

Each patient's story illustrates one or more lessons that Dr. Anderson wishes to impart *from* that particular patient's narrative to each reader. One patient learns to be observant of his body and what it is saying. Another opens to multiple possibilities for healing. Others find the courage to relinquish former beliefs; to tune into and trust their own experiences, observations, and intuition; to pay attention to how they respond to various treatments and medications; to do their own research to help figure out what is occurring and what range of treatments might be available.

I especially enjoyed the final six chapters titled *"Mysterium."*

Dr. Anderson relates fascinating stories of patient's mysterious experiences, premonitions, unusual intuitions, and dreams. His advice regarding these nonordinary experiences is wise and straight forward. "Whether the experience is rational or mysterious, at those times when we brush against the margins of reality, it is essential to pay attention." I believe that in times of significant pain, suffering, or illness, it is not unusual for people to have dreams, intuitions, or experiences that seem improbable or even impossible, but which turn out to be remarkably insightful and helpful.

Although the book made me wish Bob Anderson were my doctor, he encourages and empowers each of us to be our own best physician. He assures us that we then will be better able to work with whoever happens to be our healthcare practitioner. I love that reassuring and inspiring message.

For healthcare to move forward in the 21st century, it is important to pay attention to the lessons Dr. Anderson reveals. Be observant. Be open. Welcome change. Do your homework. Listen to what your body is trying to say. Have trust in yourself. Find out what works for you and go for it!

This book is a crowning achievement in a remarkable career. I highly recommend *Stories of Healing* to everyone who has ever been a patient. This extraordinarily insightful book will give comfort, insight, and joy to every reader.

Bill Manahan, MD

Assistant Professor Emeritus, Department of Family Medicine, University of Minnesota Academic Health Center, Minneapolis, MN
Past President, American Holistic Medical Association
Author of *Eat for Health: Fast and Simple Ways of Eliminating Diseases Without Medical Assistance*

Introduction

I am an integrative holistic medical doctor.

When I embarked on my medical career, I thought I had chosen a profession that would be fascinating, challenging, and altruistic. Little did I know that my ten years of education and training beyond a high school diploma would be just the beginning of a learning curve that has yet to make its way back to earth as I live through my eighth decade.

My medical school and internship training was *bio-medical*. My professors with their MD and PhD degrees provided me with the best information concerning what was then known about how the body works: anatomy, chemistry, physiology, microbial invasion, disease processes, deterioration with aging, and responses to treatment with drugs and surgery. I excelled in my medical education with instructors who were ranked in the top tier of highly revered leaders of their various medical specialties. In the first years of my family medical practice, as I sought to help patients, I unrealistically expected that they would all get well with the application of the superb knowledge I had acquired in my training.

Some of my patients were healed with my self-described "skillful" handling of their diseases and illnesses. Many were not. I became accustomed to hearing my surgical colleagues talk about how they healed or cured a patient of a disease by removing an inflamed appendix or gall bladder or cancerous tumor. It took years for me to realize that neither I nor any of my colleagues ever healed anyone. Healing, I finally understood, finds its origin from within the patient, from within his/her body, mind, emotions, and spirit. At best, it was my opportunity as a physician to enhance this self-healing capacity.

Many authorities have come to express this awareness in recognizing that longevity and a rewarding quality of life in our western society are determined in the main not by what we physicians do, but by what our patients do; what they eat, their exposure to their chemical environment, how they move their bodies, what they believe, and the attitudes with which they approach their daily interactions in the world. In most instances, these elements of lifestyle have an effect on life outcomes even greater than the effects of the genetic legacy gifted them from their forebears.

Through some very fortunate experiences in meticulously observing the healing experiences of many of my patients, I threaded my way through a minefield of distractions and moved beyond my excellent conventional medical training in which I dealt for the most part only with bodies. After ten years of delivering babies, checking children, treating adults, and attending the dying, I realized that I loved my work. I also became aware of my subtle re-education occurring through invaluable interactions with my patients, in paying attention to what worked and what did not work for them.

Six years into my practice, one patient in particular drew me into a new awareness of thinking about patients as whole people rather than as finely tuned biochemical machines. "Joe" came for an initial visit to my office with a classic story of a duodenal ulcer — mild heartburn and a gnawing discomfort in the upper abdomen which was relieved by eating or taking antacids. His symptoms were typically worse in the evening and better in the morning. He was not a smoker, did not abuse alcohol, and seemed to consume a reasonable diet.

X-rays confirmed the presence of his ulcer. I had treated many ulcer patients in my training and early years of practice, and prescribed the usual dietary changes and the regular ingestion of antacids — the standard treatment at the time. Joe got better. In fact, within a few weeks, he was symptom-free and gratefully relieved of his discomfort. Six months later, however, he returned with the same complaints. This time I skipped the x-ray and reinstituted his treatment. Again there was quick relief of his symptoms and I assumed he was "healed."

To my annoyance, he reappeared yet a third time several months later with a recurrence of his same symptoms. Disappointed in his failure to stay "healed," I managed to find the time to sit down with him to learn why my treatment had achieved only short-term benefits. *I began to ask about his life.* I inquired about events which held meaning for him, requiring me to spend more than the usual

2

fifteen-minute office call.

I learned that a few years before, Joe had moved from Alabama where he had spent his childhood. In his early adult life, he had been employed at the Chrysler Redstone Missile Project in Huntsville, Alabama. As that project came to a close, he secured a job in an engineering capacity with the Boeing Company in Seattle, utilizing skills he had developed in Alabama. He had moved to a Seattle suburb; his wife found employment; they purchased a modest home and sent their two children to highly-rated suburban public schools. Everything sounded like the TV series *Leave it to Beaver* with an idyllic family setting.

I asked whether he was experiencing any stress in his life. He very quickly answered "No," but then recalled a modest neighborhood controversy. Some time previously, an adjacent home had been purchased by an African American family. The new neighbor also worked as an engineer for Boeing and the two men began to car pool to work. The black family also had children of a similar age who quickly made friends with Joe's own children and the two families got along well together. There was, however, some unrest up and down the block about the new minority family.

Joe described his vague sense of uneasiness with his new black neighbors. He said "It was like I kept waiting for a shoe to drop. Nothing bad happened, but I kept thinking it *might*." We talked about the possible origin of these feelings.

Joe had been raised in a small segregated Alabama town in which blacks lived in a separate part of town "across the tracks." Schools, churches, and lodges were segregated. Many in his white community expected unlawful behavior from the segregated black population and much of the law enforcement activity in the small town focused on the black community. In a series of extended office visits, Joe and I together learned that his anxiety arose from his unfulfilled expectation that his black neighbors would behave like the blacks in his childhood, rightly or wrongly, had been thought to behave. His insight into the origins of this unfulfilled expectation of how his neighbors might behave was enough for him to have an "aha" moment. He was able to recognize and release his expectations from childhood. This had been the source of his stress. The last of his ulcer symptoms quickly disappeared and did not recur.

Joe was unconsciously asking me for assistance in caring not only for his body, but for caring about him and his *life*. This experience nudged my worldview into a broader understanding of what medical care is really all about. In many of the stories that follow, the essential lesson for me grew from finding out how my patients were moving and playing, and what they were eating, thinking, feeling, observing, believing, and for what they were praying.

I entered the world of medicine believing that as a well educated and trained physician, I would have the opportunity and duty to treat and educate my patients. *I* would be the one with the knowledge and wisdom to impart to *them*. It took me years to realize that *my patients* were simultaneously teaching *me*. I was fortunately open enough to be thinking "outside the conventional box" to be able to move beyond the rote learning from medical school.

Each event has been for me a lesson woven into a tapestry of a transformational shift in worldview. My responsibility as a physician reaches far beyond prescribing drugs to treat unwanted symptoms and surgery to remove diseased organs; it extends into the realms of engaging my patients in life-enhancing options to enable them to be fully alive in the physical, mental, emotional, and spiritual arenas of their experience.

Healing presents itself with many faces. There is no one road, no right or wrong, sometimes not even any conventional logic at all. It behooves us all to pay attention, make observations, wrestle with making sense of them, and share them with those ready to listen. Thus the path of medical progress is enhanced.

Healing and curing may not always be synonymous. A person may experience a profound healing and yet die of a cancer. A person cured of chronic hepatitis may not experience any healing at all. The vignettes which follow are not all healings; some are probably merely cures; all were important learning experiences. The depth of meaning for me varied from appreciation to profound re-education.

I believe the energy of all avenues to recovery, cure, and healing involves the potential for self-healing from within. Quantum physicists now discuss evidence for the fact that the observer influences the observation. What I report here are some of my own thoroughly appreciated observations which insistently goaded me into a profound and rewarding re-education. As you identify with these stories, I trust that they may provide insight, understanding, and a sense of meaning for you.

We will never know it all. There will always remain some inexplicable mystery about the cosmos and life itself. Most of the stories that follow have a medical flavor with nuances I hope may benefit you on your journey. The names of patients involved have usually been changed.

Section One:
Vital Nutrients

Story 1: Correcting an Irregularity

Stan, a naturopathic physician in my community, had never been a patient. We had formed an affiliation with referral of patients back and forth, utilizing his additional skills as an acupuncturist for my patients.

Stan was in his early forties when he called and asked for an urgent appointment because he had noticed an irregularity in his heartbeat. I was able to see him in our office within hours. His electrocardiogram showed an irregular heart rhythm called atrial fibrillation. In this condition the two smaller upper chambers of the heart, the atria, begin beating extremely rapidly, quivering in a chaotic fashion up to 180 times a minute, in contrast to a normal rate of about 70. The two major lower pumping chambers, the ventricles, respond in an irregular fashion to some of these atrial contractions, causing the sensation perceived by the patient as a very irregular and pounding heartbeat.

At the time, conventional treatments for atrial fibrillation included drugs to slow down the atrial rate or submitting the patient to a procedure called cardioversion. This consists of delivering a mild electrical shock in the chest region to attempt to reestablish normal electrical impulses to both upper and lower chambers of the heart. Atrial fibrillation also increases a significant risk of developing clots in the chambers of the heart due to poor emptying. These clots can occasionally be life threatening as they escape into the blood vessels to the brain, potentially able to cause a stroke. Patients now are often anti-coagulated with blood thinners to prevent this complication.

One of the drugs commonly used at the time of Stan's episode was digitalis. As I was writing a prescription for digoxin, a synthetic form of digitalis, I learned that, as a naturopath, he preferred a drug form derived from the natural whole leaf digitalis plant rather than the synthetic form. I accommodated his request and changed the prescription.

In my evaluation of his atrial fibrillation I failed to ask myself the essential question: *Why would his heart suddenly break into this abnormal rhythm at this particular time?* Leaving with his prescription,

Stan decided to also get a second opinion from a physician friend of mine, Dr. Ralph Golan. Dr. Golan was better informed than I about the effects of nutrients on heart function. After evaluation, Dr. Golan gave Stan a slow intravenous injection of two grams of magnesium. His heartbeat converted back to a totally regular rhythm in fifteen minutes!

On returning to show me what had happened, Stan's electrocardiogram was perfectly normal with a regular rhythm of 70 beats per minute.

Stan increased his food sources of magnesium, including whole wheat, wheat germ, bran, nuts, and beet greens and began taking a supplement of magnesium citrate. He had *no further episodes of atrial fibrillation* after these dietary changes.

Dr. Golan and I submitted Stan's case history to a family practice medical journal, including prints of his electrocardiograms before and after the administration of the intravenous magnesium. Here was an inexpensive intervention with great potential benefit. The only downside is that it does not help everyone. Nonetheless, our submission was rejected for publication because it "did not meet our [journal editors'] criteria."

Impressed with the simple and totally effective replacement of what was probably a deficiency of magnesium intake in correcting an abnormal heart rhythm, I eagerly involved myself in a study of nutrition which enabled me to help other patients with nutrient issues. Stimulated to delve into the magnesium tale, I found many valid published studies indicating that adequate amounts of magnesium are necessary to maintain a regular heart rhythm, and allow potassium to function normally in the heart and in the body.[1] Magnesium is an essential mineral in over 300 separate enzymatic reactions in the body and is commonly deficient in patients with heart attack, hypertension, stroke, congestive heart failure, diabetes, migraine, and kidney stones. Some authorities have estimated that up to 75 percent of people in the U.S. and industrialized countries do not have an adequate intake of magnesium.[2] Levels of potassium and sodium are commonly checked in conventional medical practice, but levels of magnesium are not. When they are, the most common test ordered is the serum magnesium, which is commonly misleading. More accurate levels are determined by doing a red blood cell magnesium test (RBC magnesium). I also learned that magnesium is lost from the body through kidney excretion when high levels of stress and tension are present. The therapeutic uses of magnesium have still not been fully incorporated into conventional medical practice twenty-five years later.

Dr. Golan's help with Stan was ironic. I had met Dr. Golan during a time in which he had been so discouraged with the limitations of his conventional medical training he considered quitting his internship. After a prolonged discussion over lunch, my influence, among other factors, persuaded him to complete his medical training. Twenty years later, he influenced me to widen my horizons into nutritional medicine.

The importance of magnesium in human biochemistry has been known for over forty years. Historically, acceptance of new ideas in medical practice has often developed at a glacial pace. After my experience with Stan, all my patients with threatened or confirmed heart attacks hospitalized in the Coronary Care Unit of our hospital received an intravenous injection of two grams of magnesium on admission. Survival of my heart attack patients was far above average. Three months before retirement, my cardiologist consultant and I were writing orders on a patient I was admitting to the Coronary Care Unit. Finishing his orders, he turned to me and said, "I've wondered for fifteen years why you always ordered intravenous magnesium for your patients on admission [to the CCU]. An issue of the *American Journal of Cardiology* journal late last year was all about magnesium. So now I know. You were ahead of your time." Acknowledging his accolade, I decided to not ask why, although he never questioned my orders for magnesium, he never asked me why I did so. There is a hierarchy at work here. Specialists do not ask family doctors why they are doing something. And curiosity often does not break through these rules of communication. Later, an analysis of multiple studies involving 4,000 patients showed a 40 percent reduction in death after heart attack by giving magnesium.[3]

Here was a lesson learned from a patient experience because I paid attention. It also involved my openness to listen to the experience of a patient who received better treatment in the hands of another physician. It would have been all too easy for me to ignore or reject the treatment of another doctor under such circumstances. Fortunately I did not.

Story 2: I'm Going To Lose My Teeth

Elaine, age 45, was talking with me as I was freezing her nine-year-old son's plantar warts. Making conversation, she sighed that she was headed to her periodontist, expecting to hear that she needed to have three teeth extracted. "That sounds awful," I said. She replied in a resigned tone that three years previously she had developed deterioration of her gums (technically known as gingivosis). A surgical procedure, intended to stimulate gum tissue regeneration, had failed, and three teeth were now loose. She feared the worst—that the teeth would now have to be extracted.

After finishing the liquid nitrogen wart treatment on her son, I asked her to wait a few moments for me to try to contact a consultant whom I thought might be helpful to her. I was fortunate enough to get through immediately to Dr. Jeffrey Bland, an internationally known nutritional biochemist, who happened to be involved in a study on periodontitis with a number of dentists in Tacoma, Washington. He kindly listed for me the nutrients which could be helpful. I gave the list to Elaine and implored her to give the supplements a try before agreeing to the extractions. The suggestions included a daily intake of:

- calcium 1.8 grams
- magnesium 400 mg
- zinc 20 mg
- manganese 15 mg
- vitamin C 2 grams
- coenzyme Q10 100 mg.[4]

She also started using a folic acid mouth rinse three times a day.[4] Noting her hapless appearance, I enthusiastically reinforced the possibility of success with exaggerated reassurance.

Her periodontist did recommend extractions. The good news is that Elaine did postpone the procedure and after about four months the teeth had not only survived, but her gum tissues had begun to regenerate and tighten up the loose teeth, while taking on a renewed healthy appearance and color. After a year, even her dentist agreed that she did not need the extractions. It was difficult for me to tell whether Elaine translated the meaning of this happy experience into any deeper understanding about the substandard nature of her nutrition. In any event, her teeth were salvaged.

Seeing this terminal situation for the three teeth reversed by addition of adequate nutritional support for her gums reminded me that good nutrition underlies the health of every organ and cell in the body. It reinforced my understanding that many damaged tissues in the body are in a state of flux and that adequate nutrients can push the equation toward reversal of disease. Osteoporosis, coronary artery disease, type 2 diabetes, gingivosis—are all reversible. And by the same token, these problems are largely preventable. All too often, we physicians focus only on intervention in disease, with little emphasis on prevention.

Story 3: Warts

I had been seeing Michael frequently as I struggled to rid him of crops of simple warts on his hands and plantar warts on the soles of his feet. The seventeen-year-old was self-conscious about his warts and had become impatient at the tortoise-like pace at which they were disappearing with my liquid nitrogen freezing treatments. The warts were so numerous that we had stopped counting them. Progress with the plantar warts was especially slow and the treatments were definitely uncomfortable.

I interrupt Michael's story to relate my experience with my own warts. For about three years in my early thirties I had been plagued with warts on several fingers—a very bad visual advertisement for a doctor! Every few days I froze them myself with liquid nitrogen at the end of my workdays after all patients and staff had left. About the same time, after noting the presence of unexplained small white spots underneath my fingernails, I noticed a 1974 letter to the editor of the *Journal of the American Medical Association* by Dr. Carl Pfeiffer, a respected authority on amino acids. In his letter, Pfeiffer linked leukodynia (white spots underneath the fingernails) to zinc deficiency. I had therefore started taking zinc supplements as a "why-not?" option. After a few months, the white spots disappeared and never returned.

Between Michael's visits to treat his crops of warts, I awakened one morning to the realization that I had not had any recurrences of my own warts on my fingers since shortly after I had started taking supplements of zinc for the white spots beneath my nails.

With this aha! in mind, I suggested to Mike at his next visit that he speak with his mother about taking a daily supplement of zinc. I suggested a dose of 30 mg twice a day. At the following visit he had not started the zinc his mother had purchased, so I contacted her to enlist her aid in persuading him to take the zinc.

Over the next three months, Mike's wart treatments progressed nicely with greatly accelerated success. The recurrences of his warts finally ceased and the last vestiges of wart tissue disappeared to his great relief. Over the next several years when he left for college, his mother told me that he had no recurrences of his warts. She also mentioned that his continuous athlete's foot fungus problem between his toes disappeared along with the warts.

Years later, I learned that zinc is a critical element in more than 110 enzymatic chemical reactions in the skin and is essential for maintaining a strong immune system. Many authorities believe warts are caused by a virus; if so, immune resistance may be critical for resisting and healing the warts. Eventually, in 2002, I found a research paper in a British dermatology journal confirming the value of zinc in the treatment of resistant warts.[5]   In the meantime, for over three decades, all my patients with warts had benefited from taking zinc.

Once again, I realized the importance of curiosity and thoughtful observation. A missing vital nutrient related to the body's resistance to wart viruses? A fact not often offered to medical students, interns, and residents. Perhaps some day it will be.

Story 4: The Non-Healing Skin Ulcer

Thore was ninety-three. He spoke halting, but intelligible, English with a heavy Scandinavian accent. He was born in Norway and immigrated with his parents to Canada as a youngster. His first visit to my office was prompted by a non-healing two-inch x one-inch ulcer on the inside of his left ankle. The ulcer had gradually developed to its present size over about two years. He had seen several doctors, but the suggested treatments, including drugs to improve circulation, had not halted the progressive enlargement of the ulcer. He had undergone treatment with an "Unna Paste Boot" to prevent motion in the skin, but this had not helped, either. Examination of the leg showed decreased blood pressure and no palpable pulses in the ankle or foot, indicating extremely poor circulation. There were also prominent varicose veins in the calf and thigh and the skin surrounding the ulcer was thin and fragile.

I found that no one had previously talked with him about his diet. Thore loved white bread, disliked vegetables, ate few nuts or seeds, and took no vitamins or minerals. This told me he was deficient in several minerals, including zinc, known to be a critical element in healing skin problems. He was too set in his ways, he said, to change his food choices to include more minerals, so I gave up trying to modify his nutrition. He did agree, however, to begin taking a daily multivitamin-multimineral supplement including 200 mg of vitamin C and an extra daily supplement of 80 mg of zinc.[6]

Thore's wife said she had heard that honey applied to ulcers was "good." I inwardly scoffed at the idea and avoided a direct answer which would admit that I knew nothing about this alleged attribute of honey. I agreed to check it out and talk with them about it at the next visit. I went the medical literature and found a score of trials using honey in non-healing ulcers. I learned that honey has an anti-bacterial effect, often clearing ulcers of infection. Further, there was evidence for stimulating healing of ulcers in which circulatory problems were playing prominent roles.[7] Thore and his wife began placing a dressing saturated with raw honey twice a day on the ulcer, lightly held in place by an elastic bandage.

After two weeks, my measurements showed that his ankle ulcer was beginning to close. I was much relieved, because his son was an internal medicine specialist in Seattle, and my treatment approach was very unconventional. After a month the ulcer began to heal rapidly and by three months it was completely closed and covered with fair quality skin. He continued the extra zinc for another three months and then stopped. He was faithful about taking his vitamin-mineral supplement until his death three years later. His skin ulcer had not recurred.

It seemed obvious that supplying Thore with zinc and the use of honey contributed to the healing of his ulcer. After my experience with Michael (story 3), I knew that zinc is an important mineral for enzyme reactions in the skin. Research studies also show that people are often lacking in zinc and that many skin problems are at least in part due to this deficiency.[8] More and more reports of the benefits of honey have been published since my experience with Thore. Taking the supplements and using the honey were clearly correlated with the healing of his two-year-old ulcer which had been progressively enlarging.

Other nutrients which may contribute to skin ulcer healing include:

- copper
- vitamin A
- vitamin C
- vitamin B-complex
- L-arginine
- adequate protein.[4]

I fortunately listened carefully to the diet that Thore and his wife described. Paying close attention to the nutritional literature describing the importance of nutrients proved critical for helping Thore heal his ulcer.

Story 5: The Rattling Artificial Hip

Judy presented in a motorized wheelchair for her first visit to my office when she was thirty-two. She had heard by word of mouth in the community that I included a wider view of therapeutic options beyond the limitations of conventional drugs and surgery.

Judy had first begun to develop joint stiffness when she was nine years old. By the time she was twelve, her attending physician diagnosed rheumatoid arthritis (RA). Appearing during the juvenile years of life, RA is often very aggressive. Her severe arthritis limited her physical activity, in turn leading to loss of bone density, or osteoporosis. The course of her disease had been steadily progressive, and about three years before seeing me, her joint deformities and physical limitations had forced her to face critical decisions about being self-supporting and being more in charge of her disease. She had returned to school, obtained her undergraduate degree, and at the time I saw her, was completing internship training prior to taking on her first job as a social worker.

Judy was single and an only child. Her support system was meager. Her parents were elderly and her circle of friends was limited.

Her inability to be physically very active had led to her being moderately overweight. Her past medical history included several joint replacements including fingers, knuckles, and hips. One hip replacement had been done on the left and she had had two replacements of the right hip. These surgical implants had kept her functioning, able to drive a specially equipped car, and maintain her ability to dress herself, prepare food, handle papers, write, and type.

Following her first right hip joint replacement, the metallic shaft of the artificial hip had become loose after about two years, due to resorption (loss) of bone around the shaft within the marrow cavity of the bone. At the second surgery the artificial hip prosthesis was replaced by one with a larger caliber shaft, tightening it within the femoral bone. The outside thickness of the femur was thinning. The successful result of the second hip replacement had held for another three years.

The precipitating issue which brought her to my office for an alternative opinion was the recurrent progressive deterioration in the right femur. Her loosening metallic shaft had begun to rattle within the bone. She had been told by her orthopedic surgeon that she would have to have a third replacement. This would be the last one she could have because the cortex, or outside rim of the remaining bone, would be too thin to sustain the pressure of weight bearing of any larger shaft.

Judy had become so depressed over the prospect of having a non-functioning hip which would greatly limit her mobility that she had decided she would commit suicide rather than face the prospect of being a total invalid. On taking her history, I was especially alert to her mineral intake since her enforced sedentary wheelchair lifestyle and inability to exercise predisposed her to osteoporosis and bone loss. Indeed, she had few dietary sources of calcium, drinking practically no milk or eating any cheese, cottage cheese, or yogurt. She also had a low intake of calcium-containing green leafy vegetables such as collard, beet greens, kale, and broccoli and consumed little in the way of seeds and nuts.

On performing an examination of her while in her wheelchair, there was an audible rattling when she moved her right leg or when I moved it for her.

Cow's milk derivatives gave her large amounts of rectal gas, abdominal bloating, and intestinal cramps. Since her history was typical for a person with lactase deficiency, I found that she traced her family history back to central Europe. Lactose intolerance or deficiency is much more common in persons of southern or middle European nationalities. This hereditary trait renders the intestine unable to digest lactose, the sugar in cow's milk. None of her doctors had addressed this problem. She took vitamin and mineral supplements only sporadically.

She agreed to avoid milk derivatives, make some gradual dietary modifications to get more calcium-containing foods, and begin to take a mega-dose vitamin-mineral preparation regularly. The supplement gave her a daily intake of nutrients the body needs to build bone, including:

rattling hip

- calcium 400 mg
- magnesium 250 mg
- manganese 15 mg
- zinc 20 mg
- chromium 200 mcg
- vitamin C 1 gram
- vitamin K 100 mcg

All these nutrients, in addition to adequate protein, are necessary to build bone. She also began taking an additional 1,500 mg of calcium daily as a separate supplement.

Over the next four months, the *rattling of the prosthesis within her femoral bone gradually ceased* as she manufactured new bone to tighten itself around the prosthetic shaft. She became less despondent, encouraged by the response of her body to better nutrition. This "aha" for her encouraged her to believe that she could be more in charge of her body and her disease.

Many authorities at the time of Judy's experience taught that osteoporosis was irreversible, but her experience teaches otherwise. Cases such as Judy's taught me that bone deterioration can be reversed and bone density improved. The medical literature now confirms that awareness.[9] Resistance exercise, a great stimulus to increase new bone formation, was nearly impossible for Judy in her nearly-wheelchair-bound status. The shift to increased consumption of whole foods and the addition of food supplements was sufficient to accomplish the task.

Story 6: Skin Deep

Practicing physicians are expected to keep up with new developments in medicine by attending seminars and reading medical journals. For many busy practitioners, this is an onerous task, falling far down the list of urgent things to do. Highly rated first-line medical journals feature research studies which are "peer-reviewed" and vetted by medical authorities before publication. Physicians also receive "throw-away" journals which feature less rigorously prepared articles that often reflect the thoughts or observations of a single author.

One day, while quickly perusing one of these throw-away dermatology articles, my attention was drawn to a short essay describing successful treatment, and indeed prevention, of cold sores and fever blisters with the use of a dilute topical solution of zinc.[10] I immediately recalled several patients plagued with recurrent fever blisters who responded poorly to the drug treatment available at the time.

Fever blisters and cold sores are caused by the herpes simplex virus. Cousins of this virus cause chicken pox, genital herpes, and shingles (herpes zoster). After an outbreak, the herpes viruses tend to remain as unwelcome residents in the body, flaring into outbreaks when the immune system is weakened by psychosocial or physical stress.

On a why-not basis, I asked my compounding pharmacist to formulate the 0.25% zinc sulfate solution for my next patient presenting with fever blisters. It worked extremely well, clearing the fever blisters in about three days. As I used this simple and inexpensive prescription more frequently, patients began to report that on applying the solution immediately after noticing the first tingly warning symptoms, which precede the outbreak, the eruptions would often be frequently totally avoided.

It happened that my mother-in-law was also plagued with frequent outbreaks of cold sores around her face. My wife began to suggest this treatment to her, in part to have some answer to her frequent complaints about her affliction. My mother-in-law harbored skepticism about a medical suggestion coming from me and it took her some time to overcome her resistance to trying it. After several episodes, she responded to her daughter's suggestions (accepted more readily than mine). She had great success and finally became a "convert," finding that prompt application with the first warning signs of the outbreak usually prevented the whole sequence.

I concluded that if my skeptical mother-in-law found this simple inexpensive prescription successful in dealing with her cold sores, it must surely be valid.

The final chapter in my awareness of the importance of zinc in herpetic problems was written some years later. I had begun to notice a small irritation in the fold between my nose and my cheek. I tried to ignore it for several days, until one night I was awakened from sleep by an intense burning quality to the irritation. The burning sensation led to my immediate conclusion that I was having a shingles (herpes zoster) outbreak. The shingles herpes virus also causes chicken pox, which I had had as a youngster. An episode of chicken pox usually induces immune resistance which lasts for several decades.

Unable to get back to sleep, I considered whether zinc would have the same benefits against the herpes zoster virus as the herpes simplex virus. Having none of the 0.25% zinc sulfate solution in our medicine cabinet, I went to my supplement drawer and pulled apart a capsule of zinc and mixed up a paste of the zinc powder with water and applied it beside my nose. Within 10 minutes the burning sensation *ceased* and I returned to sleep.

I learned from a throwaway medical journal and my mother-in-law that zinc, even applied topically, should come to mind with any non-malignant condition affecting the skin.

Section Two:
Infections

Story 7: Jacob's Otitis Media (Ear Infection)

During a "health break" at a hospital Wellness Day seminar during which I was speaking, a woman and her daughter in the audience came up to talk with me. The daughter's eighteen-month-old son, Jacob, had experienced almost continuous middle ear infections (otitis media) for over a year. His speech development was delayed as a result of impaired hearing resulting from the repeated infections. His pediatrician had referred him to an ear, nose, and throat specialist who had scheduled him for surgical insertion of ear tubes. This operation, consisting of making a hole in the ear drum and holding it open with a tiny tube, is intended to interrupt incessant recurrences of middle ear infections. Once the infections cease and a child begins to hear better, normal hearing will often be restored.

For months, Jacob had developed each new middle ear infection within four days of finishing an antibiotic for the previous episode. Jacob's mother and grandmother, however, were anxious about the scheduled procedure and wondered whether I had any suggested alternatives to the proposed surgery.

I briefly inquired about his diet and asked whether he had any allergies. The mother answered no, but the grandmother quickly reminded her that Jacob was subject to developing a rash around his mouth whenever he ate oranges or drank orange juice. Eliminating oranges when Jacob was only a few months old had cleared the rash. Shortly after that, Jacob began to have one ear infection after another. Oranges are an important source of vitamin C, which is one of the nutrients the body needs to maintain strong immunity to fight infections. So, I suggested that they start giving him a 250 mg chewable vitamin C tablet each day until I could make time in the office schedule to evaluate the child.

In prior decades, removing the tonsils and adenoids had been a popular procedure designed to reduce the recurrences of ear infections. Medical science moved on, however, and the "T &A" fell out of favor with the introduction and broad availability of antibiotics.

In about a month I did see Jacob. He had been faithfully given his daily vitamin C, and had been off antibiotics and *free of ear infections for 25 days*. The family had postponed the ear surgery. Over the next eighteen months, Jacob had only one ear infection which cleared quickly with antibiotics. At age three, he was still below the median for hearing acuity, but his tests were rapidly improving and catching up to the average.

In this instance, the addition of vitamin C to Jacob's intake appeared to make a distinct difference in the course of events. As a "why-not?" option, nothing would have been lost in trying it. Since vitamin C is important for optimal immune function, there was some logical connection to the outcome. Children with recurring ear and throat infections are known to have decreased levels of vitamin C.[11,12] The body fights infections through the production of free radical chemicals which help the body defend itself. When overwhelmed, however, excessive production of free radicals occurs. The overproduction then becomes destructive, in and of itself. Vitamin C neutralizes this excess free radical production and is rapidly consumed in the process.

Otitis media in childhood is very common, with an estimated yearly incidence of seven million infections in the U.S. Family physicians and pediatricians continue to often treat otitis media with antibiotics. In Jacob's case, he had been given 13 courses of antibiotics over the span of one year.

The immune system with its millions of white blood cells and reactive antibodies protects us against bacterial and viral invaders and snuffs out pre-cancerous growths before they develop into detectable malignancies. This remarkable immune system operates efficiently and optimally only when supplied with adequate nutrients including vitamin C, zinc, and other nutrients.

Allergic reactions also often play a prominent role in middle ear problems in childhood. They also tend to be reduced in the presence of adequate vitamin C. Vitamin C, for instance, reduces exercise-induced asthma in the allergic patient. Immune resistance in older children and adults is also weakened by unmanaged stress and a sedentary lifestyle and enhanced by relaxation practices and meditation.

An age-old debate has ensued since the time of Louis Pasteur in 1870: which is more important, the virulence and deadliness of a microbe or the immune resistance of the patient? Both affect the outcome of any infection. Unfortunately, through a combination of circumstances, our "Western" diet in industrialized countries often fails to furnish many of the nutrients essential for an appropriately resistant immune system.[12]

The addition of vitamin C was critical for the resistance of Jacob's immune system. He never knew that he helped reinforce my appreciation for the value of nutrients which are essential for the maintenance of immunity.

Story 8: "Doctor, help my sore throat"

Robert came to my office complaining of nasal congestion and an extremely sore throat. His wife and 17-year-old son both had mild sore throats. Robert had been working long hours for about two weeks on a special project for his supervisor at work. In two separate, prolonged meetings, he had been enclosed in a room where two other employees were smoking.

Robert's temperature was normal and the soft palate and throat were only mildly inflamed, significantly less than I would have expected from the intensity of his symptoms. A screening test for streptococcal infection was negative. Robert expected that I would prescribe an antibiotic. With some time-consuming explanation, Robert understood that his sore throat was being caused by a virus, in which case antibiotics would not be helpful.

As an initial treatment plan I asked him to buy a bottle of vitamin C and a package of zinc lozenges on his way home. I suggested that he take an initial dose of four one-gram tablets of vitamin C, repeating the same dose in four hours and again four hours after that. I warned him that high doses of oral vitamin C can lead to excess rectal gas, and can occasionally cause diarrhea with continuing high doses. Absent these symptoms, I wanted him to continue to take vitamin C every four hours, reducing the amount the next morning to three at a time, and later that day to two grams per dose. He was also to suck on the zinc lozenges, one about every four to six hours. In addition, I suggested a couple of aspirin tablets initially for relief of any pain which might keep him awake.

He awakened the next morning, ecstatic about what he estimated to be ninety percent improvement. He did cut back on his work schedule, tapered his vitamin C to one gram at a time over the next three days, and quickly went through the resolution of the sore throat and mild head cold.

In the medical literature, there is no shortage of conflicting information surrounding the use of vitamin C to help prevent or treat infections. Many nutritional studies and the experience of many medical practitioners do, however, support the validity of

Robert's experience. Vitamin C blood levels 24 hours after the onset of symptoms of a cold or flu can be almost as low as levels found in patients with scurvy.[4] Vitamin-C-depleted mice die from infections at three times the rate of mice whose vitamin C levels are normal. The best summary studies indicate that, at the very least, vitamin C shortens the course of recovery from viral sore throats and colds. Vitamin C has also been shown to have a broad antiviral effect, making it potentially helpful for many common viral illnesses.

In my family medical practice, each year I saw a marked increase in ear and throat infections in children around Christmas and Valentine's day. Increased intake of sugar around these holidays was probably the culprit, since processed sugar is known to erode immunity. Persons under stress are found to have markedly increased levels of free radicals and profoundly decreased levels of vitamin C. The stress of smoking leads to deficiencies of vitamin C. The vast majority of the earth's animal species make their own vitamin C without having to get it from food as humans and guinea pigs do. In species that make their own vitamin C, exposure to stress induces a *10-fold increase* in the amount of vitamin C produced.[13]

Critics might point out that the improvement may have been a mere "placebo" effect or simply a "spontaneous recovery." For Robert, his gratitude at his improvement didn't try to distinguish whether the vitamin C or the placebo effect was responsible for his recovery.

Over-prescribing antibiotics has led to the harmful evolution of antibiotic resistant bacteria. I was reminded of a leading obligation of physicians: "Do No Harm." My "aha" was that supplementing with vitamin C was an option with practically no downside risk. Robert's infection was apparently viral in nature and would not have responded to antibiotics. Vitamin C and zinc to the rescue! Perhaps getting enough C and zinc all the time would bypass having to resort to fewer rescues?

The vitamin C and zinc lozenges were strikingly helpful in Robert's case.

Section Three:
Our Toxic World

Story 9: "I can't work Because of my panic"

Tom came to me as the seventh physician whom he had seen in two and one-half years. At 31, he had first seen his family doctor for spells of anxiety, panic, pounding heart, shortness of breath, and heavy perspiration. These symptoms were not consistently related to meals or any other events that anyone had identified. He was treated with Xanax (a tranquilizer like valium) with partial relief. He was referred to an internal medicine specialist who found a normal blood sugar and diagnosed his condition as "panic attacks." Tom was then treated with a beta-blocker, a drug which slows the fast heart rate accompanying panic spells. This helped but did not relieve his anxiety and restlessness. During this time he grew steadily worse and found it difficult to finish a complete week of work at his job in a machine shop in Seattle. He saw an endocrinologist who concluded after numerous tests that his thyroid was functioning normally. He concluded that Tom's problem was "in his head" and suggested he see a psychiatrist.

Through several months of psychotherapy, Tom continued to grow worse and increased his dose of Xanax to the highest recommended levels. After being on the beta-blocker for some time, he began to have a diminished sex drive and poor quality erections, a known side effect of this class of drugs. He had also seen a chiropractor and an acupuncturist before coming to see me.

I carefully combed through Tom's history for any clues his previous physicians might have missed. Responding to my meticulous questioning, he volunteered the curious observation that he never had any bad panic spells on Saturday, Sunday, or Monday morning. He also related growing steadily worse as the week progressed, with Friday always being by far his worst day. By Saturday afternoon he had nearly always begun to feel better! He had also improved during his last two vacations, which he attributed to being away from the stress of work and heavy traffic. He had begun his job in the machine shop about six months before his panic spells began. Perhaps he was having a problem related to work—handling stress poorly—or perhaps he was reacting to something in his work environment. He described being consistently exposed at work to a variety of volatile chemical agents and solvents used in his responsibilities of cleaning various pieces of machinery.

I asked him to follow a plan which I put in writing. He was to try to arrive early at work in time to check and record his pulse, after sitting quietly in his truck for ten minutes before clocking in. I asked him to also take his pulse on leaving work after he had been sitting quietly in his truck for ten minutes without listening to his radio. He followed the suggestions and kept a written record of his pulses morning and evening. For each of the first two weeks of his records, his morning pulse rose steadily from about sixty on Mondays to eighty-five on Fridays; his afternoon pulse varied from 75 on Mondays to 105 on Friday.

I had by this time come across published medical information detailing the theory of Dr. Arthur Coca, who originated the concept of the "Pulse Test" in relation to inhalant and food sensitivities.[14,15] Other factors being equal, Coca found that sensitivity reactions to inhalant or food challenges were highly correlated to significant increases in the pulse rate almost immediately after respiratory exposure or eating.

After the second week of these consistent results I suspected that he was being exposed to toxic chemicals at work. I believed that the toxic chemical exposure, if confirmed, constituted injury on the job. Blood and urine specimens were submitted to a toxicology laboratory to identify the chemicals to which he seemed to react, but the results were equivocal and not helpful.

Still persuaded that he needed time away from work, we filed a claim for injury on the job, which was rejected by the state Department of Labor and Industries. He had accumulated scarcely any unused sick leave or vacation time. Nonetheless, I recommended a leave-of-absence. Over a six-week unpaid leave from work he improved steadily and we reduced the dose of his beta-blocker drug to the point it was eliminated. He had become habituated to his Xanax and his dosage had to be reduced very slowly to avoid the emergence of bothersome withdrawal symptoms. With the addition of biofeedback and cognitive-centered counseling sessions, he ceased having all panic episodes and decided not to return to his old job.

Was his problem stress? Six weeks with no pay plus a search for a new job were also certainly not without stress. He continued to steadily improve during this time and it appeared that his symptoms were related to exposure to volatile chemicals to which he had become sensitive. His newly found freedom from panic spells confirmed that this was an environmental sensitivity and not related to psychosocial stress.

It was essential that I spend enough time with him to provide the space in which he could report the minute details of his symptoms, so that I could help him make sense of it.

In our modern era of "Better Living Through Chemistry," thousands of chemicals have been introduced into industrialized societies. It is important to remember that most of our degenerative diseases—coronary heart disease, cancer, diabetes, brain deterioration, kidney failure—are extremely rare or completely unknown in primitive, indigenous societies. Historical studies have confirmed the rise of many of these degenerative diseases in "primitive" cultures coincident with the introduction of our "Western" lifestyle, including our chemicals.

Many of these chemicals lace our food, pollute our air, and invade our water supplies. Newspaper headlines often highlight scientific studies revealing a new chemical offender which makes people ill or causes death. Lead is found in toys from China. Chlorination of water benefits us by killing most potentially harmful germs, but combines with organic residues in water sources to form organohalides which lead to an increased level of bladder and rectal cancer in those drinking unfiltered water. Pesticide and herbicide chemicals accumulate in the fat tissue of animals and human beings. And previously unrecognized side effects of FDA-approved pharmaceuticals are known to have caused serious or fatal heart disease.

The field of environmental medicine grows increasingly more complex as our physical exposures multiply the incidence of human reactions to chemical agents.

There are no simplistic answers for contamination with chemicals, some of which are essential for vital functions in our culture. A few initial steps can be helpful:

- installing filters for drinking and cooking water;
- using high capacity filters in heating and cooling systems to improve indoor air quality;
- consuming organic food sources which can greatly reduce the detectable load of pesticides and herbicides found in the body within only a few days.

Story 10: Thrombophlebitis and Kitchen Remodeling

One early afternoon of a long work day in the mid-1980s, I received a long-distance call at my office from a 212 area code. I knew this was the area code for Manhattan, New York City, and wondered who could be calling me from the Big Apple.

Phillip was on the line. He explained that he had been browsing through a bookstore in Manhattan and was intrigued by a comment in one of my books.[16] He had tracked me down through my publisher and said he had sixteen questions to ask! Could we schedule a half-hour of my time, for which he wanted to pay me at my usual hourly rate? We found a half-hour later in the week and sure enough, he called at the appointed time. Phillip was an author's agent who lived in a high rise apartment with his partner Michelle.

The sentence in the book to which his attention was drawn was in a chapter on Environmental Medicine. It implied that exposure to formaldehyde had been reported to be a triggering factor for thrombophlebitis of the veins of the lower leg. He explained that three years before, Michelle, age 35, had experienced an episode of thrombophlebitis (inflammation and clotting of the superficial and/or deep veins of the calf). She had undergone standard conventional treatment with blood thinners, snug wrapping of the calf and eventually an exercise program. In the ensuing three years she experienced two recurrences of the phlebitis, treated each time in the same fashion. She wound up being permanently placed on anti-clotting drugs to prevent further episodes. Phillip's concern was that no cause had been found for the three episodes of the thrombophlebitis in his otherwise healthy young partner. In fact, her doctors had not probed into the underlying causes at all, but were focused only on her treatment.

Phillip began with his sixteen questions. "Do you think the total kitchen remodel in our suite, completed about six weeks before Michelle's first episode, could have contributed to her problem?" The remodeling had, of course, used standard particle board for the basic cabinet and cupboard framing. Phillip was astute enough to have read that particle board out-gases formaldehyde and other toxins for months and even years after installation. My answer was equivocal: "It's hard to say, but they might possibly have been related. It is unknown why some persons are so much more sensitive to these chemicals than others."

His final question was the zinger: "Do you think we should have the kitchen remodeled again, and require our contractor to use only formaldehyde-free solid wood, bonded with water-soluble adhesives?" I could only tell him that it was a calculated risk, with no guarantee that this was the only factor in her recurring thrombophlebitis.

Phillip wrote me about a year later that they had indeed decided to undergo the expensive kitchen remodel a second time. At the time of his writing, Michelle had had no further episodes in the year after the remodel. He then had another question. Should they ask her physician to abandon the anti-clotting drugs? Phillip described Michelle's doctor as skeptical about the formaldehyde connection. I replied by phone to tell him that I had no definitive answer, but suggested that they work with the physician to slowly withdraw the drug over a period of about three months.

Four years after the original contact with Phillip and Michelle, I contacted them while in Manhattan on a speaking engagement. They graciously hosted me at an elegant breakfast in the New York Athletic Club overlooking the south end of Central Park. Her anticoagulation had been terminated and she had had no further episodes of thrombophlebitis in the four-year interval.

As I learned with Tom, we do live in a world in which we are constantly exposed to hundreds of chemicals involved in the production of everything we use. Some of them are toxic and capable of causing serious and even fatal illness. We need to be alert to the possibilities.

It was Phillip's insatiable curiosity in asking the appropriate questions which led to a solution. These were questions which Michelle's doctor had not answered, much less asked. This is often an essential query: "Why is this [illness] [sickness] [disease] [dis-ease] happening at this particular time?" Curiosity can potentially lead to curative or healing solutions. And by then I knew enough to honor Phillip's own investigational skills in his search for answers.

Section Four:
Allergies and Sensitivities

Story 11: Outside the Box
with Rheumatoid Arthritis

Joan was 32 when she came to my office because of progressive rheumatoid arthritis of three years' duration. Joan was a stay-at-home mother of two children, devoted to her family, and working outside the home as a volunteer at school and in her church. She maintained a normal weight and had for some time maintained a program of modest regular exercise. Three years prior, in the mid-1980s, she had been referred by her family physician to a rheumatologist because of rapidly developing, progressive symptoms of arthritis. Rheumatoid arthritis (RA) is the form of joint disease thought to be due to an abnormal reaction in which the immune system produces an inflammatory chemical factor which attacks the surfaces of numerous joints in a debilitating fashion. Her laboratory rheumatoid factor test was strongly positive, and she had the typical swelling, stiffness, and pain in fingers, knuckles, elbows, shoulders, hips, and to a lesser extent in the knees. Her typical early joint deformities were distributed symmetrically on both sides of her body. In aggressive cases like hers, the arthritic process can lead to marked deformity of the hands and other affected joints, with loss of essential muscle function and strength.

She had originally been placed on a series of non-steroidal anti-inflammatory drugs like ibuprofen and at the time of her visit was on 20 mg daily of Feldene, one of the most potent ones. Later she was given tapering courses of cortisone, and was on prednisone 8 mg daily at the time of her first visit in my office. She had experienced little improvement from a series of gold injections, a conventional treatment given for rheumatoid arthritis at the time. About four months before, her rheumatologist had started her on methotrexate, an immune suppressant drug, stabilized at a once-weekly dose of 5 mg.

Joan was slowly and inexorably getting worse. She had reached the point of having to arise slowly in the morning, languidly coming to daytime functionality, significantly losing grip strength, experiencing increasingly limited range-of-motion of elbow, finger, and shoulder joints and sustaining incessant pain in all her affected joints.

On one of her office visits, while waiting for her rheumatologist in an exam room, she took advantage of the time to read about her drugs in the *Physicians' Desk Reference* (PDR) present on the treatment cabinet. She had time to read about the very serious side effects of the three medications she was taking. Her immune system was being potentially weakened by her methotrexate with increased risks of infections and possible malignancies. Her prednisone also reduced immune system function and could be contributing to osteoporosis. Her Feldene carried risks of stomach ulceration. Prompted by her alarm concerning these potentially debilitating side effects, she hastily resolved to get another opinion. Her husband, disappointed with her limitations in spite of aggressive therapy, urged her to follow through with her decision. Joan had heard that I had a broader outlook about the causes of disease, and thinking outside the box, so to speak, compared to other physicians in the community.

I went over her history, including a childhood record of allergies with hay fever and eczema. The eczema of infancy had improved significantly with the substitution of soy milk instead of cow's milk. After the age of three and one-half she had resumed drinking cow's milk with no further problems.

I reviewed the entire array of about a dozen integrative holistic options and asked her to think about which seemed most viable and practical for her to undertake. In the meantime, on a hunch, given her childhood history of cow's milk allergy, I suggested that she eliminate all cow's milk derivatives including milk, cheese, cottage cheese, yogurt, and breads and pastries, many of which contain whey and milk derivatives. I gave her a detailed milk elimination protocol sheet and asked her to follow it for fourteen days and return.

On the 11th day, she called to talk ecstatically with my receptionist, having suddenly and unexpectedly awakened that morning, free of pain and joint swelling, although her joint range of motion was still limited. As scheduled, she returned on day fourteen, markedly improved. Scarcely able to accept the abrupt change in her symptoms, she demonstrated the absence of stiffness and swelling and increased range of motion of her major joints. Her improvement was telling us that her body had responded favorably to the avoidance of cow's milk. Trying to be as scientific as possible, I asked her to confirm the apparent noxious effect of cow's milk on her joints by challenging herself with three glasses of milk daily. On day four of the challenge all her symptoms returned with a vengeance, far worse than they had ever been. She immediately again abated dairy products, and five days later her symptoms again dramatically improved.

For the next one and one-half years she remained *essentially free of symptoms* by avoiding cow's milk and cow's milk derivatives. She stopped her methotrexate at once, gradually tapered her prednisone to 4 mg daily, eliminated the Feldene, and finally tapered her prednisone dose to 1 mg daily and then stopped. This process took about eight months. She was free of pain and joint swelling at that point, and her joint range-of-motion had returned to over 95 percent of normal. I lost track of her at that time, and have heard indirectly that she was doing well seven years later.

Allergy specialists taught me in medical school that the only target organs for allergic reactions are the nose and sinuses (hay fever), the lungs (asthma), and the skin (eczema). Allergists also think that ingestant foods as a source of serious sensitizing reactions are rare to non-existent, especially in adults. Joan's experience confirmed for me what physicians espousing different medical principles (Clinical Ecologists) have long taught—that *any organ of the body can be the target for an allergic or sensitivity reaction.*[17] In Joan's case it was her joints. Her experience made me aware that food allergies and sensitivities can cause serious and debilitating problems. Reactions such as RA are usually explained by invoking an auto-immune response of the body itself. In Joan's case, the cause was an external agent—cow's milk—which triggered a sensitivity response in her immune system.

I also learned again that the human body often manifests an amazing capacity for self-healing. In her case, *the rheumatoid arthritis joint changes reversed themselves*. It would be the height of hubris to say that we can always discern how to evoke that healing. If we would but pay attention, we might be able to more often connect patients to that healing capacity.

Stories Of Healing

Story 12: "I haven't slept well since I was a teenager"

Forty-two year old Carol, her husband, and two children were patients in my family medical practice. She worked part-time as a classroom assistant in one of our local elementary schools. She came to see me with two fairly minor medical problems. When we had decided what to do about them, I observed that she looked really exhausted. She acknowledged her fatigue and said that she had not been sleeping well. Forgetting about the press of the office schedule, I discovered on further inquiry that she had not really slept well for at least twenty years.

A major problem was urinary frequency, which roused her from bed about six times each night to empty her bladder. She recalled some degree of nighttime bladder frequency as far back as high school. During the day she was accustomed to emptying her bladder at least every hour to hour and a half. Her urinary urgency during the day and at night was such that she felt in danger of wetting her underclothing if she procrastinated. Many urine specimens had been analyzed over the years with no evidence of infection. She had borne two children, but the bladder problem predated her pregnancies by several years.

On one occasion she had undergone a cystoscopy (examining the bladder through an instrument inserted through the urethra) which revealed nothing abnormal. She had never been extensively studied for ureteral reflux or kidney problems, but her kidney function tests had always been normal.

I turned to her past history in the chart. She had been allergic to milk as a child, having colic as an infant and hay fever as a youngster. I decided to postpone any further testing until she had considered food sensitivities as a possible cause of the urinary urgency and frequency. I explained my hunch, and she agreed to follow a printed food-elimination protocol which prohibited milk, corn, wheat, sugar, citrus fruit, nuts, eggs, chocolate, soy, food dyes, and preservatives. I used the protocol taken from the published work of Dr. Doris Rapp, a well known physician and clinical ecologist.[18] I gave Carol the detailed sheet of "forbidden" and acceptable foods; she agreed to try it for a week.

Three days later she talked ecstatically with my staff, reporting that she had gotten out of bed to urinate only twice the previous night, and that she was voiding at about two-hour intervals during the day. By the end of the week, she had no nighttime urination and was emptying her bladder about every four hours during the day.

The next step was to ask Carol to challenge herself with each of the eliminated foods in pure form, one at a time, at three-day intervals. Within hours of introducing wheat, and later pure chocolate, she returned to an urgent, every-ninety-minute voiding schedule during the day, with nighttime urination almost every hour. None of the other foods bothered her in any way.

Carol demonstrated a clear and unmistakable pattern. Following her discovery, she had no further urgency or urinary frequency except for an occasional episode of knowingly bingeing on chocolate.

We physicians are all too often remiss in delving into the relationship of food and micronutrient intake (vitamins, minerals, essential amino and fatty acids) to diseases and illnesses manifested in our patients. Medical schools are even now not adequately emphasizing the teaching of nutritional medicine to students. And in Carol's case, she had been the victim of a total lack of interest by her physicians in the relationship of food sensitivities to her bladder frequency. As mentioned in the case of Joan (Story 11), conventional allergists downplay the commonness of food sensitivities in adulthood and the urinary tract is not thought to be a target organ for allergic or sensitivity reactions. Moving beyond the limitations of conventional teaching and paying attention to the relationship of nutrient intake to symptoms in her case was strikingly helpful. Once Carol had been provided with the necessary knowledge, she essentially made the discovery herself.

Story 13: "It can't be mumps again"

Todd was complaining of acute, painful swelling behind the corners of his jaw and below his ears on both sides. On examination he had tenderness and enlargement of both of his parotid glands, the salivary structures which become markedly swollen and tender when invaded by the mumps virus.

Todd was 31 years of age, married, and the father of two children. He had had mumps in childhood and it would have been unusual for him to get the mumps again in his thirties. I thought he had an infection in the glands and prescribed what I thought was an appropriate antibiotic. The swelling and tenderness in his parotid glands went down very slowly, however, and in retrospect I doubted that the problem was an infection. Over the next six months he had two more brief episodes of parotid gland swelling. I referred him to our University medical system and he submitted to having x-rays taken during the injection of a radio-opaque dye into the ducts which drain saliva from the salivary glands, to rule out the presence of obstructing stones. The presence of stones in his salivary ducts could have been responsible for the swelling episodes, but the likelihood of having simultaneous stones on both sides was extremely unlikely. The x-rays were all normal and the University Clinic offered no additional options. He continued to have episodes scattered at random intervals over the next year and a half.

In the meantime, his two children, age four and six, had both shown up with sensitivity to cow's milk. His daughter's allergy presented as repeated ear infections, and his son developed recurring bouts of tonsillitis. Once milk was meticulously and totally eliminated in the children, the ear and tonsil infections ceased completely.

The experiences of his children set Todd to thinking and he recalled that his last two bouts of parotid swelling had been preceded by drinking a lot of milk. Milk had always been one of his favorite foods but as an adult his intake was somewhat erratic. I convinced him that he should undertake a provocative test of his theory.

Having eliminated all milk and milk derivatives for two weeks, he drank several glasses of milk on a chosen day and *his parotid glands began to be swollen and tender about an hour after his second glass of milk.* He repeated the challenge several weeks later with the same result. We were both satisfied that milk sensitivity was the cause. From then on, as long as he totally avoided milk, he had no further bouts of parotid tenderness or swelling.

Many allergists do not give much credence to food sensitivities in adults. Todd's experience and the preceding cases of Joan (Story 11) and Carol (Story 12) teach us otherwise. A reading of the medical literature supports the theory mentioned in Joan's story: *any body organ may be the target for a food allergy or sensitivity reaction.* The brain, leg veins, heart, intestines, joints, and connective tissues have all been shown to be targets of sensitivity reactions to ingested foods.[19]

Allergic and sensitivity reactions to foods are more common than most physicians realize. And the incidence of food reactions in the population appears to be on the increase, for unknown reasons. We physicians should more frequently think about the possibility of food reactions whenever a diagnosis is questionable or fails to be confirmed by subsequent experience.

Story 14:
"What do you mean – a five day fast?"

Kerry was 39. All the members of her family had been patients for several years. Her third and youngest child was about seven when Kerry decided she wanted to do something about her weight. She had followed a number of popular diets, successfully losing significant weight, but each time subsequently regaining it. At five feet five she did appear somewhat overweight. As we explored what was going on, it was apparent that her weight would often fluctuate several pounds in just a few days, even when she thought she had not been eating differently. She also related feeling "puffy" and felt she was "retaining water" much of the time, noticeably aggravated just before her menstrual period. Most of the time, she could scarcely remove her wedding ring.

Kerry also complained of vague, fleeting muscle pain which was often severe and centered in the front of her left chest between her breast and shoulder. She had even considered whether this might be a symptom of a heart problem. The fact that the pain was not related to exertion was reassuring, although a paradoxical variety of heart pain can on occasion be more common at rest. She was not taking any medications, so drug side effects were not a consideration.

Kerry worked as a part-time coordinator in her church, and was otherwise home much of the time managing her household and children. Her husband was gainfully employed in a job which adequately supported the family although they sometimes struggled to make ends meet. She exercised sporadically and consumed a diet which was somewhat better than average.

At the initial visit for exploring her weight problem, her left upper chest muscles were surprisingly tender on examination. Her legs were mildly swollen above her ankles ("pitting edema" in medical terms) and she had just finished her menstrual period. Her laboratory tests revealed normal thyroid metabolism and no other helpful clues; screening tests for inflammatory problems and arthritis were negative.

On checking normal weight tables she appeared to be about

thirty-five pounds overweight. She agreed to keep a journal of everything she ate for one week. When she returned a couple of weeks later, my office nurse calculated her caloric intake which was surprisingly low at about 1,350 calories per day. Having been acquainted with her over several years, I had every reason to believe that her diet record was very likely honest and accurate. As I obtained a more detailed description of her previous efforts at losing weight, it appeared that she lost weight but very slowly, and only when her caloric intake was less than 900 calories a day.

Just prior to her second office visit, I happened to have reviewed the studies of Dr. Theron Randolph, a Chicago physician who pioneered research in food allergies and sensitivities and published several papers in the 1960s and 70s. While exploring a wider array of helpful options for treating patient problems, I had followed his theory of "masked" sensitivity patterns. In these circumstances, a food reaction is accompanied by an addiction or craving with prompt and *rapid relief from symptoms after consuming the offending food*. This often leads to overeating and snacking, thus contributing to obesity.[20] According to Randolph, omission of the food offender for five days is often followed by heavy urination (diuresis), reduced swelling (edema), and sudden loss of weight.

I questioned her about her eating patterns and she did indeed describe difficulty handling periodic binges of eating certain foods. On a hunch, I sketched out a couple of possible stringent food elimination plans. One required her to eat nothing but pears, lamb, carrots, and rice for five consecutive days. An alternative protocol required her to fast with nothing but water for five days. To my surprise, she chose the fast, by far the more formidable of the two. Armed with printed materials, she left the office, determined to undertake a prolonged fast for the first time in her life. Part of her task was to record her weight every morning at the same time, and record her level of muscle pain each day.

Kerry experienced hunger and weakness during the first days of her fast. Driven by her enthusiasm and determination to explore her weight problem, she was able to cope with these symptoms.

Late in the third day of her fast, she left a message at my office.

When I called her back, she related two things which sounded very encouraging. She managed to tell me in animated language that she had already lost eight pounds; but she was anxious because her muscle pain had progressively worsened. I reassured her that both of these changes were not unusual and actually quite hopeful. A week later, at her followup visit, she appeared less puffy, noticeably thinner, and extremely happy over her weight loss of *eighteen and one-half pounds*. She had begun to pass copious amounts of urine beginning on the second day; this had tapered off but had not yet returned to normal. Her muscle pain and tenderness was all but totally gone. By the fourth day, she experienced a sense of increased energy.

She eagerly listened as I outlined the next phase of her investigation, which she managed by herself with a little advice. I assured her that the loss of edema and rapid improvement in her musculoskeletal pain was related to an allergy or sensitivity to one or more foods. When she fasted, the withdrawal of whatever food to which she was sensitive caused temporary worsening of her pain, but also soon began to let her body release the excess water. One might expect to lose about two to three pounds of weight from fasting for five days, but the loss of over eighteen pounds had to have been mostly from loss of body fluids.

Kerry then introduced the most likely food offenders one at a time, adding a new food every third day. On encountering an offending food, she could expect to quickly begin to retain fluid and experience a resurgence of her muscle pain. Over the next month, she introduced nine of the most likely offenders in this fashion (cow's milk, wheat, processed sugar, corn, oranges, eggs, peanuts, chocolate, and soy) with no hint of problems. The next group of foods included pork, one of her favorites. Only hours after she had a meal with pork, the swelling began to re-accumulate and she was aware of renewed muscle pain. It took another three to four days for her symptoms to clear. She later re-challenged herself one more time to confirm the offensive nature of pork for her. With this insight, she eliminated pork permanently.

She discovered no other significant offending foods as she completed all her food challenges. Pork *had been one of her favorite foods* and she had been accustomed to consuming it once or twice a week. In retrospect, her love of pork could have tipped me off as to its possible suspect nature. Her weight fluctuations ceased, indicating they had also been a part of the attraction/withdrawal pattern of this "masked" sensitivity to pork. Her muscle pain disappeared and her energy improved. With diligent attention to her nutrition and physical activity she lost an additional fifteen pounds, to come very close to her ideal weight.

When confronted with Kerry's symptoms, I had fortunately paid attention to Dr. Randolph's published studies. Here again, my field of possibilities was not limited to the conventional medical literature, because I had noticed the ecological studies which pursued innovational concepts. They were clearly beyond the scope of my medical school experience and training.

Too often we do something just because that's the way we've always done it. The pioneers mentioned in the afterword were keen observers about phenomena no one else had previously noticed or described. New concepts in the medical world are commonly rejected because they do not fit what we've always done.

Thinking and exploring outside the arena of conventional medical practice have often taken me out of my comfort zone and moved me several stages further into my metamorphosis of medical thinking.

Section Five:
Lifestyle Practices

Story 15: Thorvald's Winter Wood Supply

My office staff received a message requesting a house call from a family whom we had not seen before. After office hours I knocked at the door of a home only a few blocks away from my office. The house had the exterior look of a two-story structure built in the 1920s or '30s.

I entered a soundly built residence with an atrium in the center of the structure, open to both the first and second floors. In the center of the atrium on the first floor was a large wood burning stove. I could see that this was the principle or only source of heat for rooms around the periphery of both the first and second floors.

I was ushered upstairs to Thorvald's bedroom where I met a tall man who gave his age as 97. With a heavy Norwegian accent, he was able to tell me in slightly garbled speech that he had awakened that morning with great weakness in his right arm and slurring of his speech. On examination he had an obvious droop in the muscles of his face, and weakness in the major muscle groups in his right arm. His vital signs were stable. I explained that he had had a mild stroke at which point he impatiently told me that he already knew that!

I suggested that he be hospitalized, at least briefly. He resisted the idea, but with the tenacious persuasion of his wife, his daughter, and family, who arrived while I was there, he finally relented. While hospitalized, his condition remained stable and his stroke symptoms began to wane. While in the hospital, his wife and family wanted to be sure that I knew that he "worked too hard" preparing his entire winter supply of stove-length pieces of wood for their woodstove. Each fall he arranged with the local power company to deliver a couple of old power poles which were dumped in his back yard. He then spent weeks chain-sawing stove-length rounds of these utility poles, which he then laboriously split by hand into multiple pieces to be burned in his woodstove to heat the house through the winter. The family was absolutely sure the excessive strain of this heavy work at age ninety-seven had led to his stroke.

I politely suggested that the opposite was probably true: that the physical exertion had probably challenged him in a healthy way and if anything had probably postponed the time when he experienced the stroke.[21] The family was disappointed and upset that I would not urge him to give up his productive exercise. In the last analysis, nobody could have persuaded Thorvald to give up this preparation of his wood supply, anyway. He was too stubborn to accept advice from his family or from me.

I privately suggested my approval for Thorvald to go back to his woodcutting ways after recovering from his stroke. He continued to upset his family by working hard each fall and winter for three more seasons. Three weeks after celebrating his 100th birthday with fifty family members and friends (myself included), he quietly died in his sleep.

People rarely suffer downside effects of exercise; it's nearly always the opposite. I'm glad Thorvald was so determined. Physical exercise could be called wheelchair prevention.

Story 16: Seeing Is Believing

In the late 1970s, I had become intrigued with conferences offering "alternative" and "complementary" approaches to the concepts of healing. For a couple of years announcements had arrived on my desk of an annual labor day seminar at the Mission Valley Conference Center in San Diego, sponsored by the Holistic Health Association. Hearing enthusiastic reports from friends, I decided to register and attend.

I flew to California and rented a car to get about the city from my lodging on the campus of the University of California San Diego north of the city in La Jolla. I attended excellent sessions at the convention center, along with a couple thousand others in attendance.

I had also registered for post-conference workshops on the UCSD campus from Labor Day Monday through Thursday of that week. I had registered for a full complement of workshops for three and one-half days, but found nothing of interest scheduled for Monday and Tuesday mornings. Wanting to get my money's worth, I found a "Vision Workshop" scheduled for three hours on Monday morning and continued for three hours on Tuesday morning. I had no idea of the content, but it did fill out my schedule.

The workshop came at a time when I had just acquired my first set of bifocal lenses in order to continue to read fine print at a comfortable distance. About forty of us arrived at the campus classroom on Monday morning to find printed signs posted all around the room reminding us to "Blink and Breathe." The workshop was taught by Dr. Ray Gottlieb, a nationally known optometrist. Nearly everyone in attendance was wearing glasses. After an introductory lecture, Dr. Gottlieb began to work with those of us in attendance, leading us in a series of extensive eye movement exercises, looking at images on cards, and fusing images together with eyes intermittently crossing. It was initially very frustrating, since I could not see any connection with anything practical.

Finishing the first three-hour session on Monday morning, Dr. Gottlieb led us in checking the caliber of print we could clearly see without glasses. I was astonished to find that my vision had improved to the point I did not need my bifocals to read fine print at a close distance.

By the end of our workshop at noon on Tuesday, I could see clearly the finest print (comparable to four point type) without my glasses and with the page held comfortably twelve inches from my eyes. I could not deny the obvious improvement in vision. *Had I not had the experience,* I would have not believed that such a change was possible.[22]

As we left the workshop, Dr. Gottlieb asked how many of us had experienced a significant improvement in our vision; seventy-five percent of us raised our hands. We then heard Dr. Gottlieb tell us that to maintain our visual improvement, we needed to devote a half-hour each day to performing the eye exercises. As I flew back home to deplane in Seattle, I reflected on my time schedule, concluding that there was no way I could squeeze out thirty minutes each day to devote to my vision. My worldview had shifted, however, and I remain convinced that, had I found the time, I would not be wearing eyeglasses today.

Part of the explanation of the improvement stemmed from the "blink and breathe" admonitions in the classroom. I later found research showing that under stress, we tend to stare, and with prolonged visual focusing on computer and television screens, we tend to blink less often. These habits dry out and thin the mucous blanket bathing the eyeball. This shortens the effective focal length of the eye and causes visual images to fall behind the retinal surface, creating a condition of far-sightedness with poor focus for near vision.

There is scarcely anything more persuasive than personal experience. In attending this workshop, I could have verbalized many theoretical medical reasons why my vision could not improve, but these elements of denial could not overcome *my experience.* "Seeing is believing" in this case became a literal statement. My belief system had shifted again.

A number of years later, I attended a workshop on Osteopathic manipulation. Conventional medical school teaching holds that the movable bones of the infant skull become fused in late childhood, making the adult skull a rigid, unyielding bony structure. I was fascinated with lectures by Dr. Irving Korr, renowned Professor of the Texas College of Osteopathic Medicine, who reviewed his research proving that the bones of the adult skull are not fixed, but do move as appropriate. One aspect of movement occurs with the "Cranial Rhythm," a subtle expansion and contraction of the envelope of fluid surrounding the brain and spinal cord and occurring about eight or nine times a minute. In working with a partner in this workshop, *I was able to feel the cranial rhythm*. This experience caught me by great surprise, leaping over my high mountain of skepticism.

Like my Gottlieb vision workshop experience, I would not have believed it unless I had experienced it.

Story 17: He Reversed His Diabetes

A.P. was happily going along life's merry way, doing his share of overindulging and enjoying too much to eat and drink as he approached retirement. I had become acquainted with him when he attended two classes I taught for a local Elderhostel Institute affiliated with our local Community College.

At 6 feet 3 inches, A.P.'s weight had steadily increased from a mid-life manageable 235 pounds to nearly 275 pounds. On more than one occasion, he had promised himself he would go on a diet. His only exercise was a weekly game of racquetball, which caused his knees to protest because of the weight he was carrying. He persisted, however, because it was his way of getting some little bit of activity. One January, as one of his New Year's resolutions, he decided to go on another diet, which proved to be short lived. He told his co-workers he'd lost five pounds. One of his "pals" sarcastically remarked: "That would be like throwing a single deck chair off the Queen Mary." In February of that year he and his wife traveled to Scottsdale, Arizona, to visit her brother. While there, he consumed a lot of Mexican food and drank a lot of beer.

On returning home, urinary urgency and frequency prompted a visit to his family physician. He had a prior history of prostate infection. Urinalysis did confirm the presence of infection in the urinary tract, but his doctor said there was an unexpected finding: sugar was present in the urine. For some weeks, A.P. had ignored the unquenchable thirst he had been experiencing, a classic sign of diabetes. His blood sugar was well into the diabetic range with a reading of 400 mg/dl (normal = below 105 mg/dl).

This really didn't come as a surprise to him, since his mother and all of his sisters had diabetes and his nearly blind maternal grandmother had died of the disease as a double leg amputee. After the initial shock, he asked his doctor what he needed to do. He was told to get a home glucose testing kit. His physician gave him prescriptions for glyburide (a drug to enhance insulin production) and glucophage (Metformin) to improve the action of insulin in the cells of his body.

Discovery of his diabetes served as a wake up call, driving him to get serious about managing his health. A.P. was determined to avoid his grandmother's fate from the ravages of this disease. He went on a crash course to understand his disease and determine what diet might be the best for him.

At one of the classes where I met him, A.P. discussed his current health challenge with me. A friend had experienced good results with the Atkins diet and A.P. wanted my opinion. Although the Atkins diet did not seem to agree with a lot of people, given all the circumstances, I thought it might be a good choice. He purchased the book and read about the Atkins approach. Light bulbs began to go on when A.P. learned about the impact of simple carbohydrates on blood sugar control. The glycemic index was also a new discovery for him. High glycemic foods are those whose starch content is quickly metabolized to sugar. Both A.P. and his wife began to adhere to the dietary guidelines of the Atkins protocol. They also began to consistently go to an exercise facility three times a week. His blood glucose came down to manageable levels in about a month, with fasting levels in the 130 to 140 range (normal 70-105). His weight began to fall with a loss of six to eight pounds a month in spite of the fact he did not feel hungry. He felt fortunate to have caught the high blood sugar levels before any permanent damage had occurred. He had experienced mild changes in vision for a month but they ceased as he changed his diet and exercise habits.

He began to enter his weight and blood sugar levels in a spread sheet so he could keep track of his progress. He attributes this compulsive record keeping to the experience of having been trained as an engineer "to analyze everything that moves." When he had lost about 20 pounds, he was able to stop taking the glyburide and continued on a reduced level of glucophage. He had purchased a copy of a book I co-authored, *The Complete Self Care Guide to Holistic Medicine*,[23] and focused on the chapter on type 2 diabetes which suggested alternative options to prescription drugs. A.P. started taking a megadose multivitamin-multimineral supplement. This began supplying each day, among other nutrients,

- vitamin C 750 mg
- magnesium 300 mg
- zinc 15 mg

A.P. felt his energy improve when he had been on the supplements for about six weeks. Most non-pharmaceutical interventions need to be tried for at least a month to be certain about the results.

The next thing A.P. added was chromium picolinate. He began with 1,000 micrograms a day and observed the results. Within 15 days his fasting sugar levels had decreased by another 10 mg/dl, enabling him to cut his glucophage dosage in half, from 1,000 to 500 mg/day. He had been on the diet and medications for about eight months and his weight was down to about 220. He reveled in fitting into pants with waist sizes below 40 inches.

Then A.P. added cinnamon. He found cinnamon capsules on line and introduced them into his daily load of pills. Within 30 days his glucose levels fell an additional 5-8 mg/dl. Both the chromium and cinnamon worked well for him and had taken his fasting sugar levels down to the 90-100 mg/dl range. A.P. says, "My doctor was amazed when I showed him my spread sheets and he could also see a much smaller version of me in his office. *I was now nine months into my new life style and I was taken off all prescription drugs*! Diet, exercise, the megadose vitamins and minerals, and the two complementary preparations," A.P. said, "had literally made a new man out of me."

Both A.P. and his wife continued on the Atkins protocol; A.P. lost nearly 75 pounds. He was back into size 36 inch pants and wore the same suit coats he wore in college. "I felt better than I had in years." He still very carefully watched his simple carbohydrate intake and avoided any form of refined sugar. A.P. from time to time has occasionally slipped back into old routines, realizing that bad habits often lie in ambush. His renewed feelings of energy and success each time brought him back to his intention to stay healthy. "Thank the good Lord, I'm still holding my own without any prescription drugs."

I learned through A.P.'s experience that it is often essential for patients to inform themselves about the details of any given disease. A.P. paid attention to the results of each initiative he tried. He decided to take charge of his lifestyle and his diabetes, for all intents and purposes, disappeared. His glucose tolerance test after he had totally changed his lifestyle was that of a non-diabetic—completely normal! *He had reversed his disease.* A.P. was also open to trying supplements not commonly prescribed by conventional physicians.

Research suggests that up to 91 percent of type 2 diabetics can *reverse* their disease when they evoke determination to change their lifestyle.[24] Medical schools emphasize the drug treatment for diabetes such as those with which A.P. started. Drugs only change the levels of blood sugar. Lifestyle interventions can change the patient who has diabetes into one who does not have diabetes. We doctors cannot make changes *for* patients but we can facilitate the decisions of patients to make changes for themselves. That's good news, indeed, for those caught in the epidemic of this common degenerative disease.

Section Six:
Attitudes And Emotions

Story 18: Volunteering For Life

Marnie was 50 when I first became acquainted with her. Her husband held a well-paying job and she seemed to lead a happy, comfortable life. Her children were grown and within a few years of our first visit she and her husband became grandparents. Her physical health, however, was precarious. She had experienced two severe episodes of deep thrombophlebitis of the calf, leaving her left leg chronically swollen. Thrombophlebitis, encountered in the previous story of Michelle (Story 10), involves inflammation and clotting of the veins of the calf. Marnie took anticoagulants (blood thinners) for several years to prevent recurrence of the thrombophlebitis. She had also developed high blood pressure for which she took prescription drugs, and had developed early signs of coronary heart disease, with chest pain accompanying any marked physical effort. Her health was progressively deteriorating.

When she was fifty-eight, her husband was found to have prostate cancer. Two years after treatment with surgery and radiation, he was found to have metastases of his cancer in his bones and other organs. He died of his cancer about three years after its initial discovery. In his three-year struggle, Marnie was intimately involved as his major caregiver.

Marnie experienced a profound sense of loss following her husband's death. In my office about two months later, through a cascade of tears, she spoke about her sense of emptiness. She was not financially well-off, but with her survivor's income from her husband's retirement plan and her social security at age 62, she would be able to get by.

I knew that Marnie tended to thrive in being with people. Seated in my consultation room, she plaintively asked "What am I going to do?" When she gave me that opening, I suggested that finding an opportunity to do volunteer work held potential for lifting her depressed mood. I urged her to stop by our local hospital and speak with the director of volunteers before returning home.

After Marnie left, I quickly reached our hospital director of volunteers by phone, and told her that Marnie needed to be busy and would be stopping by to talk about volunteering. Our director guided her through the brief course of candy-striper volunteer training and assigned her to the medical-surgical floor where she learned the ropes of assisting the staff with a broad array of tasks. She became such an integral part of her hospital unit that the paid staff sorely missed her when she was absent. She thrived on her interactions with patients and staff and eventually expanded her volunteer time from one half-day to four half-days each week. On her volunteer days she ate lunch in the hospital cafeteria with fellow-volunteers and reveled in listening to the rumors of what was happening in the medical community and the hospital.

Marnie's health remained manageable, although she was at extremely high risk for disastrous complications. She developed further vascular problems in her calf, her electrocardiogram looked terrible, she had low-grade continuing heart pain, her hypertension remained under only marginal control, and she manifested early indications of type 2 diabetes. Her blood sugars and cholesterol tests grew progressively worse.

Over her thirteen years of volunteering, she collapsed with life-threatening emergencies on three different occasions while she was "at work" on her hospital floor. With each of these episodes, cardio-pulmonary resuscitation by the emergency team in the hospital was required to revive her. On one occasion, after having been rescued from a near brush with death, she was awakening in the intensive care unit when I reached her bedside. Her first words were *"When can I go back to work?"* Such was her enthusiasm for what she was doing in volunteer service to her hospital patients.

At an awards ceremony a year and a half before she finally succumbed to death at age 75, she was honored for her contributions as a hospital volunteer. One of her fellow-volunteers receiving the runner-up award had donated 1,500 hours of volunteer service. Marnie had donated 12,000 volunteer hours to the hospital over the previous thirteen years.

Passionate dedication to volunteer service appeared to be a major contribution to keeping her alive in spite of enormous disease problems. After her husband's death, Marnie's bleak prognosis for survival would have been limited to perhaps two to three years. In some curious and wonderful way, her joyous devotion to altruistically serving others proved to be a major factor in improving the quality and longevity of her life.

Marnie was clear that her purpose involved offering service to others, which also gave her great joy. She was unpaid in the usual sense, but exulted in her sense of importance and competence. The outpouring of appreciation came from the hospital staff and patients alike. She became a magnet for attracting others to engage in volunteer service.

Our sense of what happens biochemically and physiologically when we passionately engage in an activity we love is not well documented. Marnie's ten-plus years of unanticipated survival is the most engaging example of the benefits of passionate service which I have repeatedly observed.

Opportunities for volunteers both here in our own country and abroad are legion. Nursing homes, hospitals, and schools often depend heavily on volunteer workers to supplement their paid staffs. Great non-monetary rewards accrue to volunteers working for the needy and underserved as well as to the organizations which they serve.

In a thirteen-year study, altruistic service was identified as a primary activity related to greater longevity in aging persons, adding several years of productive life.[21] Benefits exceeded those accruing from physical workouts. Volunteerism is a prophylactic measure to maintain health and should be recognized as such.

Story 19: Giving Voice To Feelings

Helene, a patient seen in my office for more than fifteen years, came to see me complaining of diarrhea. She was 58. She had reported occasional diarrhea in the past, but it was always fleeting and never persistent enough to warrant medical treatment. Her symptoms had been present for about two weeks and I assumed that a microorganism was responsible and treated her symptomatically, expecting the diarrhea to subside quickly. When it did not, she returned, and we obtained stool samples for a bacterial culture and a search for parasites. All her tests were normal and a sigmoidoscopy found no cause for her diarrhea which appeared to have no apparent organic basis. I continued her symptomatic treatment.

Helene was a tense person with perfectionistic tendencies and I told her I thought stress might be playing a role in her symptoms. This she quickly and vehemently denied, emphatically stating that all was well at home, that she was quite comfortable with her social life, and that she had no stress of any kind. I continued to offer her symptomatic treatment with Lomotil, which remained partially successful except for occasional urgent episodes of rushing to the bathroom.

She continued to have symptoms fitting the picture of irritable bowel syndrome. She completed a clinical plan to eliminate suspected food triggers which resulted in no improvement.

About three and one-half months later she obliquely asked "If stress were a factor in someone having diarrhea, what kind of things could be involved?" We began to focus on specific details of her history, including that fact that her mother had died two months prior to onset of her symptoms. Her mother's death in her eighties was not unexpected. She had stayed in Helene's home for about three years, before finally needing 24-hour care. She was then moved to a nursing home in a community 60 miles away, close to Helene's two sisters. Helene had no particular guilt about putting her in the convalescent facility and talked quite openly about it. She appeared to have previously said her good-byes to her mother and seemed to have gone through a normal grief process after her death.

I inquired further and found that she had been appointed the administrator of her mother's modest estate. She mentioned that her sisters were uncooperative in obtaining all of the final bills, accounting for funds used for nursing home care, and in supplying necessary information for the many legal documents required for finalizing the closing of the estate. She felt frustrated by her siblings. At one point, her sisters had come to her home in an attempt to resolve the issues. She was so angry with them that she fled to the bedroom on seeing them coming, leaving her husband to deny that she was home.

As Helene talked, it became obvious that the deep resentment of her sisters was intense. Her description was accompanied by an increased tension in her posture. While relating her story she was close to tears and visibly angry. I told her that I thought the diarrhea was related to the accumulation of unexpressed frustration and that she would probably continue to have symptoms until the issue was resolved. I suggested that she verbalize her feelings, expressing her anger to two empty chairs as if her sisters were present. She was not willing to do this and the issue remained unresolved.

Six weeks later she returned, still having diarrhea. I suggested "If you can't bring yourself to talk to a couple of empty chairs, write a letter to your sisters, expressing all your past and present resentments, closing with any appreciations you have for them. Then give the letter to her husband to destroy." "Well," she said, "There won't be any appreciations." She was non-committal about her assignment as she left the office.

I did not see her for six months, at which time she came in with completely unrelated symptoms. I questioned her about the diarrhea. She told me she had finally written the letter early one morning, after which *she had no further diarrhea whatsoever*. The next day she had been motivated to write a letter of reconciliation which she did send to her sisters, eventually leading to the restoration of their relationship.

Helene unknowingly taught me that expression of intense feelings about a life trauma is usually therapeutic, when done in a safe and supportive environment. Our emotional experiences are closely related to our health and our dis-ease.

In a functional problem such as Helene's, it is often easy to remain in denial, blaming our symptoms on something else but ourselves. Not permitting ourselves to consider the fact that symptoms may be rooted in our own maladaptive thinking and emotions may require upregulating our courage to search out the truth. It was difficult for Helene to come to that realization. The unrelenting persistence of her symptoms finally forced her to address her feelings.

Hostility and anger are related to a host of medical problems, including heart disease in some of the stories which follow. Anger is a normal feeling which nearly all people experience sooner or later. When we hang on to anger for long periods of time and cannot or will not let it go, it works at its insidious biochemical promotion of all free-radical-related degenerative diseases.

Helene's epiphany with the abrupt cessation of her symptoms speaks for itself. She suddenly became aware of the connection.

Dr. James Pennebaker has pioneered the technique of expressive writing in which a person writes for 20 minutes on each of three consecutive days about her/his most significant recalled emotional trauma.[25] Extensive reports documented significant improvement in immune system function months later, and patients with asthma and rheumatoid arthritis were twenty to thirty percent better six months after their writing experience *with no other new treatment*.[26]

Story 20: Calming A Mother's Hysteria

Wilma sank heavily into a chair in my consultation room and immediately burst out "You've got to help me. I just can't go through with the wedding on Saturday!" It was Tuesday and she appeared close to panic. In her forties, Wilma was facing her role in the large church wedding of her son, the oldest of four children. I had been the physician for her and her family for several years, and Wilma's anxious behavior was hardly unexpected. She consistently experienced a high level of stress, allowing fear to crowd out rational options to solving her problems. In response to her cry for help, the only thing that popped into my head, with little conscious thought on my part, was "She has to rehearse. She needs to practice the wedding in her mind."

With Wilma seated and her eyes closed, I started my tape recorder, and began with a brief relaxation exercise taking about two minutes. I then asked her to imagine awakening on the following Saturday morning refreshed and rested, having a leisurely breakfast with her husband, having sufficient time for a relaxing soak in the tub and getting herself ready, and slipping into the new dress she had chosen for the occasion. I suggested that she imagine leaving in plenty of time to reach the church with no rush, and being met by members of the bridal party and escorted to the room where the wedding party was gathering. "Imagine warmly greeting members of the wedding party, and sense your great happiness over the joyful occasion. Experience yourself being ushered into the church sanctuary by Alex [her younger son], seeing your son [the groom] entering the front of the church with his best man, his ushers and the minister; sense yourself hearing the processional music for the approach of the bridesmaids down the aisle followed by the bride and her father."

Continuing on, I led her through images of the ceremony, the organ recessional, being ushered out of the church sanctuary and greeting the guests in a broad passageway leading to the reception hall where brunch was to be served. I suggested that she would remember the names of everyone coming through the reception line, warmly introducing them to the rest of the wedding party. I followed with images of her making guests comfortable at their tables at the brunch, playing the role of the gracious hostess. Bringing her focus back to my consultation room from the wedding fantasy, I gave her the tape recording and suggested she play it as often as she could in the five days before the wedding. I accompanied it with strong reassurances that everything would go well.

Some two weeks later, she returned to the office on another matter. I asked how the wedding had gone for her. She related that the entire day had gone exceptionally well and she had been relatively calm. She volunteered that she was very surprised she seemed to recall the names of guests in the reception line she hadn't remembered that she knew. On questioning, she said she had re-played the tape recording forty times between Tuesday and Saturday morning.

The stress of anticipated situations can frequently be minimized by imagining a sequence of positive events happening the way we would wish them to take place. The influence of Wilma's imagined experience on her nervous system and emotions was a powerful reaffirming "aha" for me.

The human nervous system does not distinguish between perceived reality and imagination. We can awaken from a frightening dream with a feeling of panic as powerful as if we were experiencing it in reality. The nervous system gifts us with emotions consistent with the content of our imagery of an upcoming event. Repetition reduces the stress of any given experience, whether real or imaginary. The forty-first time that Wilma experienced the wedding sequence was much easier than the first or second time she did it in her imagination.

Athletes, amateur and professional alike, often rehearse their performance in their own mind's eye. Their achievement is usually enhanced in so doing. Dr. Roger Bannister, the first runner to break the four-minute mile in 1954, practiced his event and trained his body for only 45 minutes each day. But prior to breaking the record, he is said to have often gone to sleep at night imagining completing his one-mile run, breaking the tape and hearing the timer say 3:59.9.

Use of the imagination was not taught in my medical training. I was fortunate enough to have enrolled in post-graduate seminars in contemporary psychology and counseling in which imagery and visualization were taught as effective means by which we can help accomplish the changes we choose to make. I had already begun to use that awareness in appropriate clinical situations before Wilma challenged me with her hysteria.

Section NINE delves further into the use of the imagination.

Story 21: Grieving, Forgiveness, and Liver Disease

In the early years of my family medical practice, the two families in this story began to establish their primary medical care with me; the fathers of the two families were identical twins, Larry and Lenny. It was a joy to have these families in my practice, because their worldview had a serious side which had made them aware of the importance of their lifestyle in maintaining their health. Both families faithfully practiced their religious beliefs, which meant that they did not smoke, drank no alcohol, and made healthy food choices. Patients with healthy lifestyles always made my task much easier.

Larry and Lenny worked in the asphalt paving industry. They had both acquired great skill in running the giant machines which can roll out an absolutely smooth asphalt surface on a highway that is being paved or repaved. Their exceptional skills placed them in great demand in the industry and they were able to provide very well for themselves and their families. Larry and Lenny were extremely close. They fished together, hunted together, and played together. They had remained so similar in physical appearance that I had continuing problems in telling them apart.

In his early forties, Lenny died from an apparent heart attack, suddenly, and without warning. There had been no prior signs or clues in his history, physical examinations or screening blood tests. Larry experienced a flood of emotions on his brother's death: grief and sadness; anger at his brother for leaving him; and anger at God for "letting this happen." Over the next years, Larry tried to substitute as a surrogate father for his nephew who was two years old at the time of Lenny's death. He experienced bouts of depression, and his laboratory tests showed compromised liver function. To no avail, I searched for the source of his deteriorating liver tests; he drank no alcohol, was not overweight, and had not been knowingly exposed to any liver toxins. In retrospect, he may have had chronic hepatitis C, for this occurred before hepatitis C was widely recognized as a medical entity. Without a specific diagnosis, there was then no definitive treatment for his deteriorating condition.

Larry was in need of counseling for his depression and volatile emotions, and he agreed to see my wife, Joann, a trained mental health worker in our medical clinic. The death of his brother still weighed heavily on him every day. Larry had made no progress with his depression and had lost his zest for living. I knew serious psychological work would be necessary to let go his bitterness over Lenny's death. The subtle fatigue accompanying his progressive loss of liver function also contributed to his depression. Both Larry and I were alarmed at the downhill slide in his health from his progressive liver deterioration with no real hope for recovery.

The series of counseling visits with Joann began about ten years after Lenny's death. Larry's nephew by then was twelve years old. This boy had been the 'apple of the eye' of both twin brothers and they had big plans for taking him hunting, teaching him to fire a rifle, and learn the nuances of being an excellent fisherman. When Lenny died, the boy's "fathering" fell to Larry.

In the fourth session of working with Joann, Larry broke down for the first time and cried and cried and cried over the loss of his brother. Then he talked out his anger, went through the act of forgiving his brother for dying and forgiving himself for not being with his brother when he died. He had believed he might have helped save his brother's life had he been present with him at the time of the heart attack.

In his next to last session, he exploded with great rage at God. Joann set out the highest chair in her office and had him stand on the seat of the chair to play the role of God. Larry and his "God," by switching roles back and forth, had a long conversation, during which time he finally forgave God, releasing his demands that God should have kept his brother alive and should have taken from his shoulders the burden of caring for his nephew. His facial features displayed immediate relief from his stress and his body language marked him as being in a very different 'space' when he left that day.

In his last session he was happy as a lark and excited about spending more time with his nephew. He had numerous activities planned. A few months later, a recheck on his liver functions showed *75 percent recovery toward normal*. His energy and enthusiasm returned and he had no occasion to be seen in my office for several years.

During his counseling sessions, Larry shifted several of his beliefs: 1) that he could have prevented his brother's death if he'd been there; 2) that God could or should have prevented his brother's death; and 3) that substitute-parenting his nephew was a burden. There was another distorted belief, too, that he changed: that his brother died on purpose to avoid raising his son, leaving the parenting to him. Of course that was nonsense, given what we knew about the family. Forgiveness is often the last therapeutic intervention which can restore energy for life, love for self and others, and the realization that one can still find a new purpose in living after being struck by tragedy.[27]

Medical science has shown that what one believes profoundly affects outcomes. This, of course, is known as the placebo effect: belief alone can be a factor in healing. I have more than once thought of having a bumper strip designed to say *"You have to believe it to see it."*

Story 22: Asthma:
Emotions Run Amok

A call from the Emergency Room of my hospital alerted me that a patient of mine had arrived by aid car. She was described as being in "status asthmaticus." This is a condition occasionally occurring in persons with bronchial asthma, in which the constriction of the breathing passages is so extreme that the air exchange in and out of the lungs is marginal enough to be life threatening. The usual bronchodilating drugs are ineffective and often the condition mandates insertion of a breathing tube into the windpipe.

By the time I arrived at the hospital, an endotracheal tube had been inserted and she was being managed by a pulmonologist, a specialist in respiratory disease. I had little to add to the treatment, but obtained a detailed history from her husband who was dressed in paint-splattered coveralls.

Over the span of a decade, Gertrude had come to the office intermittently for minor conditions. Occasionally we had the opportunity to talk about her asthma, but she managed her disease rather well by herself, utilizing only bronchodilator inhalers. She was a diminutive wisp of a woman, weighing less than one hundred pounds, and her husband was over six feet tall with a large frame. She and her husband were in their early sixties; I had occasionally seen them together and recalled some tension in their interactions in my office.

During the early evening, she and her husband had been repainting their living room walls. She was painting the lower portion of a wall and he was painting with a roller near the ceiling while standing on a high step-ladder. She noticed that he had dripped a large blob of paint on the natural-finish base shoe and had spilled paint onto the rug.

She immediately flared into anger, screaming and raging at him for doing such sloppy work, not noticing the spill and demanding he climb down from the ladder immediately to clean it up. Within minutes she was markedly wheezing, her asthma in full expression. A few minutes later, as her air exchange became alarmingly limited, her husband called for the aid car. Her struggle to breathe became so extreme he became frightened that she might die before the medics arrived.

I asked if he had previously ever observed such a severe asthmatic attack triggered by anger. He recalled similar incidents of serious loss of air exchange with severe wheezing, but nothing approaching the threatening nature of this episode.

The story ended with her full recovery from the episode after five days in the hospital. Following up in the office, I judiciously approached the role anger had played in the episode. She was in some denial about the incident, but admitted, "I did let my anger get out of control." She was not, however, about to deal with the issues underlying her predisposition to express anger so violently.

It was quite apparent that the unbridled and extreme expression of her anger triggered the asthma "attack." Acting out her anger in such extreme fashion was life-threatening for Gertrude.

Some years later I read a newspaper account of a woman who had made arrangements for the graveside memorial service of her deceased father. Arriving at the cemetery and discovering that the grave for the casket had not even been dug, she became extremely angry at the mortician who had failed to complete the preparations. After screaming at him in a rage for about two minutes she had collapsed and died, in spite of the best resuscitation efforts of a 911 response team that happened to be nearby.

Grief and sadness, anxiety and fear, and anger and rage are normal and potentially powerful emotions. Failure to express powerful feelings in some acceptable way can also be detrimental to health, but prolonged uncontrolled expression can also be life-debilitating and even fatal. Some reasonable balance may be the best approach to survive and thrive.

Story 23: Insight From A House Call

Donny and Angela were four-year-old twins. They were the children of one of the families in my medical practice, although I had never seen the mother or father as individual patients. When their mother brought them for the first time, it was because of their asthma. New in town, she sought continuing care for the twins who had shown up with wheezing at about age two and one-half. The twins were outgoing, responsive children. They responded to inhaled bronchodilator medicine and for weeks at a time were free of wheezing. Other than the asthma, they seemed quite normal, their growth pattern was well within the norm, and their well-child checkups raised no other concerns.

My office staff received a call from the mother in mid-morning on a Monday. She had no transportation to get to the office and asked if I could make a house call. The twins were wheezing badly and she was concerned that the medicine was not adequately relieving their symptoms. The office schedule was very tight and we informed her that it would be the end of the day before I could see them at home. We asked her to call sooner if their condition deteriorated.

Reaching their home at about 5:30 p.m., I found a much-relieved mother who said that the twins' breathing had gotten progressively better as the day wore on. They were playing with great energy and enthusiasm. More to legitimatize the house call than anything, I dutifully examined both of them, finding no wheezing or obstruction with their breathing. I did not see any reason to change their medication, and made preparations to leave.

As I moved toward the front door, I became aware of a subtle sound in another part of the house that reminded me of the opening of an automatic garage-door. Within seconds, both twins start to audibly wheeze. Within a minute the father appeared; I had not previously met him. He was visibly irritated, berated his wife for asking for an unnecessary house call, and emphatically stated that the children were o.k.

The mother reached for the inhalers for both of them, and the wheezing began to subside. I suggested an increased prophylactic schedule of inhaler use to try to prevent the wheezing, rather than simply responding to the symptoms. As quickly as possible I made my exit. As I left, I was aware that I had not put much energy into looking for the causes or triggers of the asthma, but simply focused on the treatment.

This house call taught me about some of the dynamics of bronchial asthma. Had I not seen the family in the setting of their home, I would have missed the opportunity to see the interactions among the family members. The arrival of the father at home clearly triggered the wheezing response in the twins, whose emotional reactions were obviously part of the picture. In subsequent visits, the mother was unable to respond openly to my suggestion that there was an unresolved issue in the dynamics of the relationship with her husband and children.

Within months, the parents were divorced. I saw the twins but seldom for their asthma until they moved from the community about a year later. After that, I learned to always attempt to find out why a particular patient has a particular illness at a particular time.

I was not taught in medical school the value of a house call. In my span of practice, several times each year I responded to requests for house calls, nearly always gaining crucial insight by directly monitoring my patients or their family in the setting of their home. Not infrequently, observing disorganized, unhygienic, and sometimes chaotic circumstances, I realized that what I had expected my patients to do was far beyond their capabilities.

The house calls, with the benefit of objective observation of my patients' home surroundings and the impact on their health, resulted in a shifted emphasis in the way I worked with patients. I am sure it improved the quality of my medical care.

Story 24:
"I could never be good enough"

Jared and members of his family became patients in my practice when he was in his late thirties. Jared had a mildly increased blood pressure and was plagued with incessant anxiety and nervousness. He described being productive at work and earned a good living. He enjoyed his family, including his three children, and he and his wife relished a circle of good friends. He tried to convince me that everything in his life was harmonious except that his anxiety and blood pressure were persistently problematic.

After a number of office visits failed to shed much light on what might be contributing to his hypertension and chronic anxiety, I suggested that he join an on-going men's growth group which met with me twice a month. The men met to work on a variety of issues which were interfering with a more robust experience of physical, emotional, and mental health. Jared came with some reticence at first, but slowly adapted and became comfortable with the other men.

I had experienced working in group sessions and realized benefits in my own life which I had not gained from one-to-one contact with doctors and therapists. Well-structured groups provide a setting where group members can learn from each other and gain the sense of social support which is an important factor in exuberant health.

In my men's group setting, each man was free to "have the floor" and work on issues which surfaced as they reflected on their lives and their daily experiences. Jared slowly began to share some of his childhood experiences in which he described frequently feeling guilty because he could never seem to do things well enough to please his father. He described his father as perfectionistic and prone to criticism of him and his siblings on a regular basis. He recalled that there was always something every day that he or his siblings had failed to do, or do well enough to avoid some judgmental lecture from his father.

After Jared and his wife were married, they lived in our community not far from his parents. They began the habit of dropping in to visit Jared and his family every Sunday after attending church. Jared and the family came to dread these visits because they felt compelled to work frantically on Sunday mornings to clean and straighten up the house and yard to please his parents during their impending visit. But no matter how intense the preparation, the parents, particularly his father, always found something to criticize. The floors could be cleaner, the books should be put away, the windows needed washing, the rugs needed cleaning.

As Jared described these horrendous Sunday mornings, the other men in the group began to offer advice about the wisdom of letting the family be themselves and let his father's criticism roll off without taking it to heart. Jared tried, but the drive to please his father was too deeply ingrained to simply let go his emotional responses to the words of criticism.

In our next session, Jared's anxiety was particularly noticeable. He described the previous Sunday's experience. Having frantically worked the whole weekend to have the house perfectly prepared, and thinking that there was *nothing* his father could criticize, Jared quoted his father, "Jared, you missed a blade of grass when you trimmed the lawn next to the driveway." *A blade of grass!*

I asked Jared if he was ready to let this issue go completely. "I wish," he answered. I asked him to sit facing a vacant chair and to imagine that his father was sitting in that chair. "Your father can't say anything to you because he's only here in your imagination" I said. "Now imagine that you are five years old and feeling badly that he has criticized you for not doing something perfectly. Tell him how you decided that you would always try hard to please him and how awful it felt when he was never satisfied." Jared found the words to express this to his imaginary father. "Now," I said, "knowing what you know today, that you can never do everything necessary to avoid your father's criticism, take that awareness back to your five-year old self and tell your father that you are no longer going to struggle to try to please him because it is simply impossible. Tell him that he will just have to be critical if he chooses, but that you have decided that you will do what's reasonable and no longer engage in the obsessive struggle to please him since it won't work anyway." Again, with some difficulty, Jared found the words to express himself in the first person, speaking directly to the image of his father in the chair.

Jared *immediately* looked more relaxed and less anxious. His face revealed a faint smile. The shift was so pronounced that all of the men in the group noticed the difference. We then role-played an interchange with one of the other men in the group acting as his critical father, so that Jared could rehearse the words he would later use, including the statement "Dad, we're not perfect here, we can only manage what's reasonable."

Later, Jared reported that at his parents' next visit, he had gently pushed back. He then endured another lecture from his father, who abruptly left their home with his mother. The regular weekly Sunday-morning visitations ceased! To Jared's great relief and that of his family as well, visits with the parents became less frequent and more comfortable. Jared's blood pressure fell to a normal level and his anxiety relented, reappearing occasionally with other stressful experiences.[28] With the help and support of his group members, Jared learned that he could stop being boxed in by his habitual response to his father and allow him to have whatever feelings he had to have. Life moved on for Jared and his entire family. We rarely have to live on and on feeling totally "stuck" with circumstances we cannot change.

My medical school did not teach me that the stress of striving against impossible odds is a cause or contributor to high blood pressure. Neither did it instruct me how to help patients encounter devastating behaviors spilling over from childhood experiences. Jared's nervous system was continually on guard to try to please his father and his blood pressure was revved up as well. Finally, Jared had the opportunity to *practice a better response,* knowing that he could *never* be good enough to please his father.

His father came from a generation that believed criticism alone was a valid approach to helping an offspring achieve success in life. Psychologists, psychiatrists, and counselors have fortunately moved beyond the narrow confines of these restrictive beliefs.

Section Seven:
Doing The Research

Story 25: A Social Isolation Syndrome

Paul had taken a relaxation and stress management class from me when he was in his early 20s. When he was 42, he tracked me down to eagerly relate the striking details of his story, which I recorded in 2004. He had never been a patient and we had not seen each other over the intervening twenty-two years.

Paul had been raised in a dysfunctional family with two older sisters. There had been a lot of fighting between his older siblings and between his parents who divorced when he was 12. His mother married again, to a man who turned out to be an alcoholic.

Around the fourth grade, Paul began to manifest problems with poor focus and concentration. Later, in high school, he began noticing mental and physical exhaustion in late afternoons and evenings, feeling tense and anxious and experiencing pressure sensations in his head.

Paul was a spindly kid who had great problems gaining muscle mass. His blood pressure was found to be mildly elevated by the time he started into puberty at age thirteen. He also recalled being aware of excessive salivation and a metallic taste in his mouth after visits with his dentist; both of these sensations became progressively worse over time. He developed a condition known as "geographic tongue" with cracking, fissuring, and bleeding of the tongue surface. The salivation was so pronounced he found himself swallowing about every fifteen seconds. Becoming aware of this odd behavior, his peers inflicted incessant teasing and ridicule on him. Bullied into isolation, he had no one with whom he could share his confusion. His mother and alcoholic step-father were emotionally uninvolved in his problems. Paul began to experience serious symptoms of stress and often had foreboding thoughts. During puberty, his fears raised so many questions and self-doubt he finally persuaded his parents to arrange counseling with a psychiatrist. These visits proved to be of no benefit.

Other symptoms which he occasionally experienced included tightness in his throat and neck, a feeling of instability which he described as dizziness, ringing in the ears, and chronically cold extremities with numbness in his hands and feet. He sensed himself restricted by a sense of fatigue, never quite developing the energy of his peers.

School work was severely affected by inability to focus and pay attention. His social life failed to develop because of his sense of embarrassment over his inability to relax, his incessant salivation, and his preoccupation in attempting to disguise these symptoms. Pervasive distress over the fact that he seemed so different from his peers led to waves of anxiety which became a daily experience. Through all his remaining school and college years and young adult life, he felt immobilized, worrying about revealing his weirdness to anyone else. He later saw a counselor at Iowa State College who concluded he had profound mental and emotional problems.

Paul managed to finish high school, after which he worked at a local YMCA and enrolled in a local community college where he earned his two-year Associate in Arts degree. He then followed his old boss to Iowa State College where he earned a B.S. degree in engineering. He had since been employed in positions utilizing his engineering skills. By 2004, he was working as a grading and engineering supervisor for Snohomish County near Seattle.

He developed interest in vocal music in high school, and had learned to play the electric bass guitar while in community college. This musical interest provided one oasis of enjoyment in his otherwise anxiety-ridden, bleak existence.

In his search to find a cure for what he thought were problems of his own making, he read numerous self-improvement books, introspectively working on his own mental state and attending various classes. Nothing seemed to make much difference. In 1994 he stumbled onto a book by the controversial dentist, Dr. Hal Huggins, *Its All in Your Head.*[29] In this book, Huggins details his experience and theories about the noxious nature of the mercury used in silver-mercury amalgam dental fillings. The Environmental Protection Agency classifies mercury as a toxic metal for humans and animals.

Responding to case histories detailed by Dr. Huggins, Paul began to be suspicious about the possible toxic effect of his own fillings. His multiple dental cavities in childhood had required the attention of his dentist who treated them with application of silver-mercury amalgam fillings starting at age ten. He recalled his dentist's reluctance in placing this type of filling, but because they were the least expensive, they were used at his parents' request. By the time he finished high school he had twenty mercury-amalgam fillings. He broached the possibility of mercury toxicity with his dentist who discounted the concept and ridiculed him for entertaining the thought.

Paul contacted Dr. Huggins' office and obtained the name of a dentist in his community who was open to the theory of mercury toxicity. This new dentist measured the electrical currents generated in the mouth by the fillings. Documentation of electrical currents in the mouth is a standard part of the Huggins protocol. One of Paul's fillings generated a current of 40 microamperes, a markedly elevated reading. The total of generated electrical currents in his mouth was over 300 microamps, with normal considered to be below 10. He decided to have his fillings removed. In an extensive procedure, his dentist removed, in one sitting, the two quadrants of fillings generating the highest negative currents (approximately one-half of his fillings), replacing them with composite materials.

During the night after the removal of the first fillings, Paul awakened to a new and unaccustomed feeling of total relaxation. His excess salivation was gone. He approached his former dentist to share the joy over his improvement but met only ridicule. Paul noticed that a multitude of symptoms, to which he had unconsciously adapted, also disappeared after this first session of amalgam removal. The pressure sensations in his head were no more. His feelings of anxiety and fear faded. He was aware of more energy than any time since early junior high school. His blood pressure returned to normal. The negative thoughts were gone. The geographic tongue condition vanished and he noticed a newly found ability to gain muscle mass. He developed a sense of direction about his life and was able to focus attention on his own goals. He regained courage and confidence, and began to approach his work and social life with a heightened sense of self-esteem.

Paul believes his problems were caused not only by the toxic effects of mercury, but also by the constant negative electrical potentials generated by the metals in his deteriorating fillings.

One case never proves a theory. The American Dental Association adamantly maintains that mercury amalgam fillings do not cause toxic problems. Paul's story, nonetheless, is dramatically impressive. Combined with the stories of many others, it appears that mercury is toxic and detrimental to a susceptible subset of the population. It warrants serious consideration by those whose symptoms have not been reasonably diagnosed and satisfactorily treated by more conventional approaches. My own view is that most of us might well ask our dentists to use alternative materials for deteriorating mercury-amalgam fillings which require replacement. It could be considered a why-not option.

I was in awe of the reading and research that Paul did for himself in achieving remarkable success in overcoming obstacles to cure. The potential for successful healing was extraordinarily enhanced in the presence of this informed patient. Here again, although I never treated Paul, I became aware of the importance of encouraging patients to do their own research.

Story 26: The Meticulous Research of a Diabetic

Stephan was found to have type 1 diabetes at age 15. He was a patient of one of my family practice associates. I first met Stephan when he was 35, while his own doctor was away on vacation. Type 1 diabetic patients require insulin for their survival and Stephan had, for some time, been giving himself injections of 80 units a day. Even with this dosage, his diabetes was still poorly controlled, and he frequently spilled large amounts of sugar in the urine. He frankly admitted to having been cavalier about his diabetic control for years.

About two years before his initial visit with me, however, he had become motivated to learn more about his disease. One great factor causing Stephan to get serious about his disease came from the observation of deterioration of the retina (retinopathy) by his ophthalmologist. His eye doctor told Stephan that he had developed small retinal hemorrhages which would require laser treatment within a year and would, nonetheless, eventually lead to blindness. The appearance of retinopathy, kidney deterioration (nephropathy), and reduced nerve function in the limbs (neuropathy) are three cardinal signs of serious complications of type 1 diabetes.

Driven by fear in response to the ophthalmologist's prediction, Stephan began checking his blood sugars four times a day with a drop of blood from finger sticks. Normal readings would be below 105 mg/dl before breakfast. His tests were running over 400 mg/dl regardless of the time of day. He began to follow his diabetic diet faithfully. At his office appointment with me he brought with him a six-foot scroll of butcher paper on which he had plotted a graph of his four-times-a-day blood sugar readings for over 700 days! Never had I seen any patient so motivated and meticulous in record keeping.

Stephan had dedicated himself to his own research and experimented with different diets. He found that the high-fiber, high-complex-carbohydrate, low-fat, moderately-low-protein diet promoted by Dr. James W. Anderson of the University of Kentucky[30] seemed to give him the best control. He began to have insulin reactions on assuming this diet, forcing him to gradually reduce his insulin dosage to prevent them. After his blood sugars improved to the point that all his readings were below 200 mg/dl, he began to read about vitamins and minerals which play roles in diabetes. He exhaustively researched options in the local University Health Sciences Library. He began to take a regular supplement of multivitamins and minerals at Recommended Dietary Allowance levels. On further research, he began to take larger doses of vitamin C, beta-carotene, and vitamin E. Stephan then soon added additional minerals and vitamins, eventually consuming the doses in the bulleted list. He found a mega-dose multivitamin-mineral preparation combining many of the ingredients, with the rest taken individually.

Stephan's daily supplements:

• vitamin C 12 grams
• beta-carotene 15,000 IU
• vitamin E 1,200 IU
• chromium 200 micrograms
• manganese 15 mg
• zinc 75 mg
• vitamin B1 50 mg
• vitamin B6 50 mg
• vitamin B12 400 mcg
• biotin 8 mg
• inositol 500 mg
• magnesium 400 mg
• omega-3 fatty acids 2 grams
• alpha lipoic acid 1.2 grams
• L-carnitine (an amino acid) 1.5 grams

As he increased his intake of supplements, his blood sugar control further improved and very slowly he decreased his insulin dose to eighteen units daily. At this point all his blood sugars were running between 100 mg/dl fasting and 170 mg/dl after meals (normal = below 150 mg/dl). His daily insulin dose had dropped from 80 units a day to eighteen. His improved diet and supplements had greatly *improved* his blood sugar control while he was *reducing his insulin* dosages about 80 percent. I had been aware of research finding that substantial numbers of Americans are deficient in many vitamins and minerals, and I was glad to be able to reinforce Stephan's conclusion that supplements had been quite helpful for him.

Meanwhile he had been visiting his eye doctor every three months. His ophthalmologist reported steady *improvement* in his retinal blood vessels over nine months to the point he told Stephan that the necessity for laser treatment was no longer present. His eye doctor told Stephan that diabetic retinopathy is not thought to be reversible and *any* improvement in the retina following the onset of micro-hemorrhages was quite unusual. Stephan asked the ophthalmologist if he was interested in how he had achieved the improvement, and the doctor seemed curious. "When I explained my program, however, the ophthalmologist rolled his eyes, declaring that the supplements had nothing to do with the improvement, and stormed out of the room."

Most would concede that his improved blood sugar control would result from strict adherence to a good diabetic diet. The unusual improvement in his early diabetic retinopathy was the result of his superb blood sugar control in conjunction with high doses of nutritional supplements. Stephan was healthier and his vision and retinal function was preserved. At the very least, the time when his condition might deteriorate was greatly delayed.

We tend to think of medical research as the province of highly paid persons in white coats working in the sterile environment of a university laboratory. Clinical research is also done on a daily basis by primary care physicians and specialists *and consumers of medical services.* When we find that something works, we incorporate that something into our lifestyle.

Other patient-directed initiatives, which aid in diabetic control, include weight loss and physical exercise (see Story 17).

Many patients with chronic disease problems can aid in their own treatment by learning about their condition and *making decisions which potentially enhance their health.* For example, patients have discovered that if they learn to meditate, their chronic sources of pain are less bothersome and their dis-ease problems become more manageable. Patients who use the power of suggestion and imagination to focus on the positive aspects of their lives usually do better (see section NINE). When I began regular exercise in my thirties, my mood improved, my energy improved, and my family said I was easier to live with. With this observation and reinforcement, my personal research on exercise morphed into a life-long habit.

Not all health information is created equal. Even invalid sources can be found on the world-wide web. Stephan had spent days at a time in the medical school library doing his own research, combing through the peer-reviewed medical literature. He then applied it to himself and found that it worked.

Section Eight:
Afflictions Of The Heart

Story 27: "I can walk better"

Leonard was 56 when he was referred by a Boeing Company doctor who thought he needed a second opinion with which I could help. He related the following story.

About eight months prior to his first office visit with me he had finally capitulated to the investigation of a pain in his left calf which came on while walking. This pain had subtly begun about two years before and had progressed to the point he could not ignore it. It began to interfere with his work at Boeing and with his part-time work as a real estate agent. He could no longer walk more than two blocks on the level before having to stop to rest and allow the pain to subside. The diagnosis spoke for itself: intermittent claudication from peripheral vascular disease (PVD). The blood flow to the arteries in his left leg was severely compromised by atherosclerosis.

His physician had referred him to our University Medical Center where he was seen in a vascular disease clinic. He was told by both a resident physician and an attending physician that no pulses could be felt at the left knee, ankle or foot. He was told that his circulation would get progressively worse, and when severe enough, he could be referred for by-pass surgery to reestablish blood flow around the blockage. He was given an appointment to return in six months for rechecking.

He accepted this sentence, and shortly thereafter, while visiting his brother in Southern California, fell to talking about his circulatory problem. His brother had been to see an attending physician at the Pritikin Center in Santa Barbara. His brother insisted that he see his own physician before returning home.

The Pritikin Longevity Center had been established in 1975 by Nathan Pritikin,[31] a nutritionist and longevity researcher. Persons with advanced medical problems typically stayed in residence at the center for a month, adhering to a vegetarian diet and walking for exercise.

The Pritikin Center physician, among other things, reviewed Leonard's lifestyle. Leonard was a smoker; he had a heavy drinking habit; his diet was high in fats and sugar, low in fiber and almost completely devoid of vegetables; he scarcely exercised at all except for an occasional round of golf, now abandoned because of his leg pain. His brother's physician outlined a program of exercise and dietary change, and assured him it would likely help his circulation and reduce the pain in his left leg.

On his return to Seattle, Leonard made some tentative beginnings at starting the suggested lifestyle program. Limited to walking only two blocks before being stopped by leg pain he was forced to retire from his position at the Boeing Company.

Leonard came to see me in my office. On examination, I could feel no pulses at the knee, ankle, or foot of either leg; his feet were cool and pale. In addition to the information he had shared with his Pritikin physician, he revealed that he harbored great anger toward his first wife, who "took me for all I was worth" in a divorce settlement. He had married again very quickly, and found that the relationship with his second wife had soon become very contentious. He was also angry with his body for making his life so physically uncomfortable. Leonard was unable to find acceptable ways to express his intense feelings about these circumstances, and felt trapped in his present relationship. Leonard also expressed great anger at the University physicians who had not even hinted that there might be some steps that he could take to improve the compromised circulation.

I sensed that he needed to let go all this anger. I suggested that it was imperative that he forgive his physicians, his wives, and his own body. My suggested plan for him utilized an unusual definition of forgiveness: canceling his demands that his university physicians "should" have told him what he could do to improve his circulation, and that his body "should" not be giving him so much pain. It was important for him to understand that this cancellation of his demands be undertaken *in his own self-interest.* The forgiveness in this approach dealt only with the demands within his own mind and it could be utilized even if the person(s) on whom the demands were focused were not physically present with him.

We then tackled the continued anger and hostility harbored toward his ex-wife. I would not repeat the words he used to describe her. In spite of considerable difficulty, but motivated by self-interest,

Leonard embraced the forgiveness protocol in canceling his demands on the university physicians and his ex-wife. He *immediately* felt significant relief.

I worked with him to make as many lifestyle changes as he was able to initiate and pursue. He reduced his cigarette smoking by about 50 percent. He also was not ready to definitively deal with the emotional stress and the hostility of his present marriage and did not succeed in altering his alcohol consumption very much, either. He did, however, become motivated to make some nutritional changes and begin an exercise program, which he found much easier than contemplating changing his attitudes. He made it convenient to schedule a regular swim time five days a week, and began to walk on a regular basis. At first, his swimming was limited by leg pain to four laps in the pool. He began to swim his four laps of the pool until stopped by pain, rest until the pain subsided, then swim another four laps, continuing this sequence for about 45 minutes. When walking, he stopped at two blocks, rested for about five minutes, walked for another two blocks, alternating this walking and resting for about 40 minutes several times a week.

He modified his eating. He was accustomed to consuming most meals away from home, in part to avoid the disagreeable relationship with his wife. He changed his pattern, avoiding fast-food restaurants, and favoring those with salad bars. He deliberately began consuming less beef and pork, eating fish and poultry instead. He switched to brown rice and whole wheat bread and stopped his intake of donuts, sweet rolls, candy bars, colas, and sugar in his coffee. He made little change in fruit and vegetable intake, but did manage to increase intake of foods high in magnesium including whole grain breads, nuts, and seeds. Magnesium enhances circulation throughout the body.

At his visits to the office over the next months, he reported faithfully staying with his exercise. A year into his program, his swimming tolerance had increased to forty laps in the pool and walking *two miles* without having to stop. He was obviously delighted with his progress, and I was impressed with his dedication to his healthy initiatives.

Leonard subsequently moved from the community, and I had

no further contact with him. I had no laboratory or objective studies to prove that his circulation improved, but clinically the improvement was unequivocal. The pulses at the ankle and foot still could not be felt, but his feet were warmer and pinker.

His most important lifestyle change came with walking and swimming. He found in them the most feasible ways to activate his body. His occupation as a real estate broker provided him with a flexible schedule and opportunities for frequent exercise. It also provided him an outlet to express some of his intense feelings in the form of physical activity. With his dietary shifts, he increased his intake of magnesium, fish oil, and vitamin E, all of which improve circulation.

With his improvement, I learned that success does not depend on doing everything perfectly. It was important for him to be able to express his angry feelings and let go of much of his hostility. Being able to share that and work through it with me was obviously enormously helpful.

Even though Leonard did only part of the recommended lifestyle changes, his pain was relieved and even more importantly, *he was empowered by the awareness that he had some influence over his disease.* Vascular bypass surgery can relieve symptoms, but does not deal with the causes of the compromised circulation. Addressing causes can lead to basic changes in the life of a patient beyond merely changing symptoms.

Story 28: George's Angina

George was 49. I recall that he happened to come to see me at the stern insistence of his supportive wife and family. George stood about six feet two inches tall and had blond hair just beginning to yield to gray. At his initial evaluation he described uncomfortable sensations ("but not pain"!) in his chest with physical exertion. A resting electrocardiogram of his heart showed changes typical of severe circulatory problems consistent with coronary artery disease. I referred George to a cardiologist who interpreted his electrocardiogram as showing evidence of a previous mild heart attack, although he had no conscious recollection of such an event.

He was mildly overweight, moderately depressed and resistant to his wife's pleadings to improve his health. In the era before coronary bypass surgery was an option, his cardiologist and I asked George to make a number of lifestyle changes, including modifying eating habits, engaging in physical exercise, and learning and practicing relaxation techniques. I discussed this with him, suggesting that he would benefit from modifying his attitudes to reduce his heart disease risks.

George was a classic example of the type A personality described in the 1970s by Drs. Rosenman and Friedman.[32] Their studies correlated an increased risk of coronary artery disease with personality traits of "hurry sickness" and hostility—to which they applied the term "Type A." Ever resistant to the suggestions of others, George's thinly veiled attitude of hostility toward life remained unchanged. He decided that physical exercise was the only option he could undertake.

Over the next three months, his heart pain grew worse. In spite of vasodilator drugs and nitroglycerin for acute episodes of angina, he had to stop more and more frequently while walking because of chest pain. He worked in an office in downtown Seattle, and parked his car on the Elliott Bay waterfront. This required a short walk up three very steep blocks to his office building. At one point, George told me that in his climb to his office he had to stop to rest 24 times to allow his pain to subside before going on. His counting of his rest periods further convinced me that he was a type A.

George finally agreed to enroll in a medically-monitored community-based YMCA exercise program. His initial evaluation showed a very poor treadmill electrocardiogram and physical performance, well below average for his age. He began his three-times-weekly exercise program of calisthenics and walking on an indoor track. At first, because of his chest discomfort and shortness of breath, he was able to walk only two slow laps around the indoor track without stopping. Six months into the program, he was able to slowly jog the indoor track for twenty laps without discomfort and with little shortness of breath. He felt enormously better and greatly encouraged. By then he was able to walk up the three steep blocks to his office with no heart discomfort except on very cold mornings.

As with the previous case of Leonard (Story 27), George would not allow himself to follow all of my suggestions. He did what he could. The exercise alone, without addressing another options, was sufficient to greatly improve his angina. He remained comfortably functional for many years. It was important for me to learn the benefits of a treatment program which fell far short of the ideal. I re-experienced the aphorism "half a loaf is better than none."

George didn't have to do everything right to improve his condition. When coronary artery disease patients make this kind of progress with exercise, at least one of five things is happening:

- the heart and skeletal muscles may be taking up oxygen more efficiently
- the coronary artery atherosclerotic blockages may be regressing
- the heart muscle might be developing new collateral blood vessels to supply areas of deficient oxygen supply
- the lungs may be exchanging oxygen more efficiently
- the blood may be flowing more freely because the blood platelets (important in forming blood clots) are less sticky.

Whatever the mechanisms involved, George was greatly

improved and he and his anxious wife were delighted with his increased walking capacity.

With each decade of life, our bodies age. On average, between age 30 and 80, we lose 60% of back, arm and leg muscle strength; ligament strength declines 50%; we experience increased propensity for injury to muscles, ligaments and tendons which require longer healing times; joint cartilage tends to deteriorate; and our bones exhibit decreased resistance against fracture.[33]

A balanced program of regular aerobic and resistance exercise greatly retards the progression of all these markers of deterioration of the physical body. We all need to "just do it."

Story 29: Treating Hypertension

John had mildly elevated blood pressure. It gave him no symptoms and revealed itself in the process of a routine physical exam. John was a 38-year-old slightly built man, who, on further rechecking, had blood pressures consistently 145-150/90-95 mmHg. He went through the exercise of checking pressures at home to rule out "white coat" hypertension, for which he was a good candidate. White coat hypertension describes the tendency for some patients to anxiously raise their blood pressure only in the presence of a health professional dressed in white. John's home readings, however, were not significantly different from those in my office. Significant stress was a part of his history, resulting in part from his occupational demands as a high school teacher. He was clearly an intense man, and was easily categorized as a typical "type A" behavior person, encountered in the history of George in story 28.

Hypertension is thought to afflict 75 million Americans, over half of whom are not aware of their problem. Hypertension plays a role in heart attacks, strokes, and heart failure, taking an enormous toll in disability, death, and cost of treatment. Many physicians would elect to use a drug to reduce the elevated blood pressure found in John's case. Diuretics were the drug of choice for initial drug treatment of hypertension at the time I was working with him.

At a medical conference about a year before seeing John I had listened to an Emeritus Professor of Medicine present a surprisingly holistic concept. He had been a former Dean of a Medical School and chief of the Hypertension Clinic at his University for nearly 20 years. He emphasized that maximal efforts should be made to lower the blood pressure to normal by making changes in lifestyle. He presented impressive evidence that lowering pressures, presenting at 170/105 mmHg or lower, by means of prescribing drugs, *did not prolong life*. The serious complications of using drugs canceled out the benefit of lowering the blood pressure which should have resulted in decreasing the risk of stroke and heart attack.

John eagerly expressed interest in my suggestions for pursuing lifestyle changes instead of starting on drug treatment. The most appealing options were biofeedback and meditation. I asked him to read *The Relaxation Response* by Dr. Herbert Benson[34] and *How To Meditate* by Dr. Larry LeShan.[35] He later returned for the first of two biofeedback sessions. Biofeedback is a medical technique in which a physiological function—pulse, skin temperature, muscle tension—is continually monitored, with second-to-second results fed back to the patient. Having explained to John the theory of relaxation and biofeedback, he cooperated well in the 10-minute exercise which I tape recorded for practice at home. Much to our amazement, wile he was comfortably seated with his eyes closed, listening to my voice and quiet background music, his skin temperature rose 13ºF. When any relaxation process is successful, the nervous system reorganizes its function so as to send out fewer nerve messages to the blood vessels, allowing them to relax and open widely. With less resistance, blood flow through the relaxed vessels increases, giving off more heat from the body core and raising the temperature of the skin.

The session consisted of suggesting that John consciously begin breathing slowly and moderately deeply, exhaling slowly, and inhaling only when necessary. These initial instructions were followed with suggestions encouraging him to relax the shoulder and facial muscles and silently repeat affirmations of being relaxed. I next invited him to imagine himself visiting a quiet, beautiful, peaceful, warm meadow, falling into as deep, relaxing sleep, and then finally returning to his awareness of the room in which he was seated.

John began to engage in a daily morning practice of ten minutes of this deep relaxation. He later began to study a form of meditation, which he continued for about four years. At his periodic office visits, he appeared more focused and relaxed but still alert. Within a month his blood pressures had begun to fall toward normal. Within four months they were consistently at 125/90 in the office and slightly lower at home. One year into his program he had essentially stopped doing the original relaxation/biofeedback exercise and was following a programmed set of suggestions from his meditation study. His office blood pressures were consistently at or below 115/75 and he reported an occasional post-meditation home blood pressure reading as low as 95/50.

His resting pulse rate, about 72 at the beginning of treatment, gradually fell, dropping as low as 40 per minute when fully at rest. By that time he was also undoubtedly benefiting from many other nutritional, exercise, and attitudinal lifestyle changes to which credit should also be given for decreasing his blood pressure and pulse. The effect of his relaxation and meditation training enabled him to be in substantial *voluntary control* of his blood pressure all the time, even when he was not giving his conscious attention to relaxation..

The lesson I learned from John could be described as a maxim, "lifestyle changes first, drugs later." It would have been acceptable for me to prescribe a diuretic for John when he first appeared with his high blood pressure. But it was better for me to work cooperatively to help him modify his lifestyle. Drugs would have only changed his blood pressure. *Engaging in his relaxation procedures changed not only his blood pressure, but changed his life.*

Story 30: "I'll do anything
To recover from my heart failure"

I waited at a table set for three in a restaurant in Ojai, California. On seeing Audrey and her husband, Al, coming through the door, I stood to alert them to my presence. Audrey, the 65-year-old wife of a retired business executive slowly made her way to our table while leaning heavily on her husband's arm. Panting for breath, she sank quickly into the chair which I pulled out for her. It was fully two minutes before she could catch her breath and raise her arm to shake my hand and whisper a greeting.

Earlier in the day, I had met Audrey's husband at a quarterly board meeting of a non-profit foundation headquartered in Southern California. It was my first meeting after my election to the board in 1992. At a break in the morning session, Al had privately mentioned Audrey's heart disease and asked if I could talk with her. I suggested that the three of us have dinner together.

In 1986, Audrey's doctors had diagnosed congestive heart failure caused by cardiomyopathy. In this condition, the heart muscle fibers lose some of their ability to contract, compromising the heart's ability to perform its pumping function. She had struggled through nearly six years of increasing swelling in her legs and progressive shortness of breath on exertion and on lying down flat at night. Average life expectancy with cardiomyopathy is about two to three years from the time of diagnosis, and she had already survived for over five years.

Audrey's left ventricular ejection fraction (LVEF) had been recorded at 11 percent prior to treatment in 1986. The LVEF is a measure of the efficiency with which each stroke of the heart pumps blood into the aorta; normal is 60 percent or better. Maximum drug treatment had improved her LVEF to 25 percent, but her condition had again been progressively deteriorating for the past two years. A second opinion had confirmed her cardiomyopathy after undergoing an echocardiogram, coronary angiography and electrocardiograms at rest and during exercise. She had also developed "secondary asthma." Profound shortness of breath limited her to climbing only five steps at a time.

She was taking fourteen prescriptions. Each day she took digoxin, lisinopril, Lasix (a diuretic), potassium, Quinaglute, and Hydralazine for her heart; Seldane, Theodur, Intal, Albuteral, and saline mist with a nebulizer plus oxygen for her shortness of breath; aspirin to prevent clotting; ranitidine to counter the stomach effects of aspirin; and Premarin for post-menopausal symptoms. She had to sleep partially sitting up in bed. Her life was totally centered on her debilitating symptoms and her schedule for taking all the medications. She was able to practice meditation on a daily basis, but physical exercise had become an impossibility.

She and her husband asked if I had any suggestions for augmenting her present cardiac care. Her downhill course allowed me to be comfortable in sketching out some "why-not" options which I knew would not interfere with any of the treatment plan her cardiologist had outlined. At the restaurant table I wrote out a list of several additional possibilities, including increasing her potassium, and adding daily supplements of magnesium, taurine, and carnitine ("non-essential" amino acids), coenzyme-Q10 (a critical energy compound produced by the body), beta carotene, and vitamins E, C, and B1. I also suggested the addition of a megadose vitamin-mineral preparation to guarantee adequate intake of other antioxidant vitamins, including B-complex elements at two to ten times the Recommended Daily Allowance (RDA), plus an array of essential minerals at one to four times the RDA.[36]

At our next board meeting three months later, Al told me that Audrey had conscientiously followed *all* my suggestions and was noticeably improved and *able to climb a full flight of stairs*. Three months after that, she had just returned from an air flight to Florida by herself, managing two moderately heavy pieces of luggage. On visiting her cardiologist on her return, her left ventricular ejection fraction was greatly improved! She wrote to me:

"My doctor is amazed at how well I'm doing, and has started taking me off most all of my meds for coronary problems. Last echo [echocardiogram] showed ejection fraction of 58 percent! So - o – o, now he's interested in what vitamins, minerals and enzymes I'm taking, as you suggested. (He has a couple more cardiomyopathy patients who are not doing well and are on conventional medications). Interesting development! Thank you for your care, your heart, and your competence! Very truly yours, Audrey M. P.S. Don't know if it's attributable to vitamins/minerals etc., but I am able to perspire for the first time in my 65 years (unstuck my thermostat!)."

In the ensuing year she slowly went completely off all her prescriptions except Lasix which was reduced to one-half her previous dose. These changes were made with either the suggestion or consent of her cardiologist.

At age 77, fifteen years post-diagnosis and nine years after initiation of her nutritional and amino acid supplement program, her left ventricular ejection fraction was even better according to an e-mail from her husband in 2001.

"Docs can't figure out how her heart managed to heal—ejection rate gone from 11 percent to 75 percent !! No one can explain it, but no matter. She has allergies and runs short of breath, cannot walk a distance without stopping and resting, but otherwise excellent . . . Now that's healthy ! Stay well, Al"

By the time Audrey and I crossed paths, I had learned that levels of magnesium, coenzyme Q10, vitamin B1, and the amino acids, taurine and carnitine, are commonly very low in patients with cardiomyopathy and congestive heart failure.[36] It made sense to replenish these deficiencies with supplements. I was grateful that I had noticed this research.

Audrey also relied heavily on her strong sense of spirituality and her daily meditation. I am sure that these factors helped maintain her heart function, even at its low ebb. Rarely do patients survive for long with left ventricular ejection fractions below twelve percent.

Audrey finally succumbed to the physical deterioration to which we are all heir, dying at age 81, having survived with her life-threatening cardiomyopathy for 19 years.

Audrey taught me that not all physicians understand the nuances of nutrition and food supplements. Her steady recovery after implementing the program was impressive and persuasive and reinforced my innovative treatment for congestive heart failure patients. Nutrients, especially in concentrated form as supplements, can have profound effects. Even in life-threatening situations, the human body retains a capacity to evoke self-healing.

Audrey survived, and in a real sense, thrived, for over 19 years from the time of her diagnosis. She enjoyed a high quality of life, enabling her to do the things she chose to do, even as her life progressed into what is called "old age." Audrey and I both had to think beyond our conventional medical limitations.

My inexorable medical transformation was continuing.

Section Nine:
The Power Of Imagination

Story 31: Imaginary Desensitization

Doug was thirty-seven when he began to be plagued with worsening allergy symptoms. His mother had told him that as a bottle-fed baby he was very colicky until he was four and one-half months old. In childhood he had mild seasonal hay fever which was treated symptomatically with antihistamines and decongestants. He had never been tested to specifically identify his allergens. In young adulthood he became used to a life of using nasal sprays during the spring and summer and managed reasonably well with this minor inconvenience.

Beginning three years before I saw him, he had noticed intensifying hay fever symptoms including frequent sneezing, nasal congestion, and occasional episodes of shortness of breath and wheezing with colds and respiratory infections. The wheezing had recently become persistent. On specific questioning, he also gave a history of increased stress stemming not only from pressures of a new role at work but also the conclusion of a contentious divorce from his soon-to-be ex-wife.

Skin testing showed reactions to spring and summer pollens, dust mites, mold, and dog and cat danders. His history raised a question of a possible contribution from milk allergy. His infant colic reminded me of the connection with cow's milk intolerance in childhood. While providing additional medicine for relief of his symptoms, I mentioned the possibility of using imagery to improve his symptoms. He was interested enough to try, and a visit to record an "allergy walk" was scheduled.

Arriving for the next appointment with some anxiety, Doug was connected to a biofeedback device with a thermistor (a temperature sensor) taped to one of his fingers to feed back a continuous reading of his skin temperature. Doug was then led through a series of relaxation suggestions, starting with closing his eyes, breathing slowly, quietly and rhythmically, relaxing his shoulders, and relaxing his facial muscles. I asked him to silently suggest to himself that his body was relaxed, emotions calm, and mind quiet. I asked him to imagine visiting a quiet meadow on a warm day, listening to birds singing, seeing brilliantly colored wildflowers and sitting down in a patch of lush grass and leaning against the trunk of a tree near a clear, burbling stream, and feeling his arms and legs warmed by the sun and allowing himself to fall asleep. My biofeedback device recorded a marked increase in skin temperature, indicating he had achieved a state of deep relaxation.

I then suggested that he would drift off into a dream, finding himself first on a farm where all varieties of domestic animals are present, playing with the dogs and cats and freely breathing deeply without congestion or wheezing. I asked him to move his awareness of being on another farm where flowers, grasses, weeds, and trees are blooming and filling the air with pollen, in the face of which he finds himself breathing fully and freely with no congestion. I continued: "Then find yourself in an industrial park with the heavy stench of pollutants, petrochemicals, and volatile solvents while you breathe freely and deeply. Visit an old abandoned Victorian house in the basement of which you find mildew growing on concrete walls and wood partitions with a deep layer of dust covering all surfaces and find yourself still breathing fully and easily. Move your consciousness to visit a department store with a myriad of pungent odors of perfumes, leather goods, detergents, mothballs, cleaners, and other pervasively out-gassing products while breathing freely. Move on to a banquet hall in which you find a long buffet with an extensive display of foods of all kinds, while sampling a tiny bit of each, all the while breathing perfectly normally. And, finally, enter a large room and find within all the people whom you have ever disliked, greeting each one and genuinely wishing each of them well, moving from person to person until all have been recognized, while you breathe comfortably, quietly, and fully. Now let yourself reawaken to the sights and sounds of the peaceful, warm meadow, lingering for a while, and finally leaving to slowly return to your awareness of the room and the chair on which you are seated and opening your eyes."

Doug's finger temperature had risen 14 degrees Fahrenheit in the twelve minutes of the imagery exercise. The temperature increase was consistent with a state of relaxed consciousness and a decrease in sympathetic nervous system activity to minimal levels. I recorded the exercise on a cassette which I asked Doug to replay at least once a day at home. He took the matter seriously and after about four weeks found he could recall the entire scenario without needing the tape. The "tape" was now in his head, and he could "play" it quickly at any moment of his choosing.

As weeks and months passed, his wheezing gradually subsided and he was able to slowly decrease the use of his medicines, gradually limiting their use to only the times when his allergic symptoms flared with acute respiratory infections. His nasal congestion, too, improved, and except on rare occasions, he was free of the cycle of hours of partially obstructed breathing requiring the use of his nasal sprays.

This appeared to be a successful result of an unconventional therapy. Doug was ecstatic about the results, the best of which was his "aha" that the power of his own mind could affect changes in his body. He was motivated to continue to reinforce his progress by repetitive practice, and as time passed, apply imagery in working on other physical issues.

Not long after this story came to a favorable conclusion, I found corroboration in a study of thirty healthy volunteers who were recruited for research in the power of the imagination to affect the body. Healthy volunteers were divided at random into two groups. Each was carefully tested for the strength of the tiny muscle in the palm of the hand that brings the little finger from a fingers-spread position to touch the fourth finger (the abductor digiti minimi muscle). Group one was asked to actively exercise the muscle fifteen minutes a day by pulling the fifth finger in to toward the fourth finger against resistance supplied by the other hand. At six weeks, the muscle strength had increased 29 percent. Group two was asked to spend fifteen minutes a day *imagining* that they were forcibly pulling the fifth finger in towards the fourth finger against resistance. Their average increase in strength was 23 percent.[37]

Imagination, especially evoked when one is in the relaxed state of mind, is a largely untapped resource in the matrix of healing and maintaining health. The state of the immune system, the guardian of our resistance against invading bacteria, viruses and the development of cancer, has been shown to be profoundly influenced by the imagination.[39]

With Doug's successful management of his allergies, I learned once again to think outside the box to create a more coherent holistic medical view of healing.

Story 32: "I can't fly"

Gloria was in her early forties. She was divorced and the mother of two children now grown and out on their own. She held a clerk-level job for a Washington State agency. With careful management of her income she was able to live a simple existence and manage a mortgage on her modest home. I saw her for yearly checkups, but she was seldom ill. I did sense that she felt isolated and enjoyed only a small circle of friends.

In early fall I saw her name on the schedule for a late afternoon appointment. The note on her chart at the exam room door said she wanted help with stress. Within a few moments I had the full story.

Some weeks before, she had dropped her name into a receiving basket in a local branch of a supermarket chain which was sponsoring a chance to be selected for an all-expenses-paid one-week trip for two to the Virgin Islands in the Caribbean. She had been notified four weeks before that she was one of the three winners. She had made arrangements to get time off work for the trip and persuaded her sister to accompany her. She had, however, procrastinated facing her great dilemma: she had an intense fear of flying and a pervasive fear of heights, technically known as aviophobia and acrophobia.

Some years before she had been scheduled to fly from Seattle to California with a stopover in Portland, Oregon. Panic-stricken the entire 45 minute flying time to Portland she had gotten off the plane in Portland and did not fly on to California. So here she was, two weeks from anticipated departure to the Caribbean and panic-stricken even thinking about flying. The prospect of her sister as companion was not sufficient to quell her anxiety. As she explained her dilemma in my exam room, she grasped the arms of her chair with white knuckles. She wanted help.

I told her with a calm demeanor that we would do some mental rehearsing, and that I thought she would improve sufficiently to be able to go on her flight. As we engaged in further discussion I learned that she had great difficulty driving over high bridges. She avoided the Interstate-5 Freeway Bridge high above the Lake Washington ship canal in Seattle, and drove far out of her way to cross the waterway over the much lower Fremont Bridge.

I chose to record her entire trip, in advance, in her imagination. I started by asking her to recall a place and time earlier in her life in which she had experienced joy, warmth, companionship, and the beauty, and quietness of nature. She decided to focus on a wilderness cabin on a lake which she had often frequented with her parents and sister in childhood.

I asked her to close her eyes, breathe slowly and quietly, take herself back to her childhood cabin, identify with the feelings, and renew them in her mind. "Imagine how it felt." As her white-knuckle posture eased, I then suggested that she listen to my description of the upcoming vacation trip, and that anytime she began to feel anxious that she raise her index finger on her right hand. Beginning with driving to the airport from home, as we got to the I-5 Freeway Bridge, she raised her finger. I asked her to then go back to the cabin in her mind and lower her finger whenever she was re-experiencing the comfortable, relaxed, joyful feeling she recalled as a child at the lake. She soon lowered her finger. I guided her in her car up and over the Freeway Bridge interrupted by two more trips back to the lake cabin.

In some detail, I led her through thoughts of finding her flight at the airport, boarding her plane, feeling the plane taxi toward takeoff, and feeling the surge as the powerful twin engines lifted the plane from the runway. She had to return to the lake three more times until she was fully airborne in her imagination at 35,000 feet.

At her stopover in Atlanta we had several lake interruptions before she found her flight to St. Thomas. Getting her off the ground in Atlanta was easier, and by the time she arrived in St. Thomas, her nervous system had begun to adapt with diminishing anxiety. I hustled her through her "marvelous" week's vacation in two or three sentences and brought her back home in her imagination with far fewer interruptions.

I asked her to plan to listen to the 30-minute audiotape recording as often as she could in her remaining two weeks, and suggested that she call me on her return to apprise me of how well she had managed the trip.

Gloria called on returning home and explained that the trip went well; some anxiety emerged, but her retreat to her childhood lake worked well. She was still not certain that she would voluntarily fly again, but expressed great relief that she was able to negotiate the trip. And she actually had a good time in the Virgin Islands.

Successes like Wilma's experience at her son's wedding (Story 20) and Gloria's vacation trip are based on the principle that the mind and brain do not distinguish between perceived reality and the imagination. In fact, the same brain structures that are activated with a given activity as shown on functional Magnetic Resonance Imaging (MRI) also are activated when that same activity is imagined. Repetition, whether real or imagined, reduces anxiety, as we saw in Wilma's fear of her son's wedding.

Story 33: Unexpected Wisdom From Within

Mildred, at age fifty, was in her sixth year of crises. She experienced multiple problems, including weight gain, feelings of anxiety, panic, and depression, disappointment in her family, disappointment in her sex life, insomnia, fatigue, confused thinking, and fleeting paranoia suggestive of psychotic illness. She had seen numerous counselors, psychiatrists, and physicians of many specialties. She had not seemed to make headway in controlling her many problems. Mildred was extremely bright, mother of four children, and a talented musician. Her husband was supportive but seemingly not able to help meet her substantial emotional needs.

I had seen Mildred for a number of different medical problems and had agreed to help her work on some of her psychological issues as well. Her previous psychological work had enabled her to recall a childhood in which she was raised by parents of extremely rigid religious beliefs. She had endured pervasive verbal abuse by her mother and acquiescence by her father. There had also been physical abuse in the form of extreme spankings and being punished by confinement to a chair for hours at a time.

In the context of working on some of her issues, we turned to her problem of insomnia and poor rest as a possible cause of her fatigue and exhaustion. The insomnia manifested chiefly as a problem getting to sleep; once asleep, Mildred did not awaken through the night. Early in the discussion, Mildred happened to spontaneously mention that if she lay down for the night before 9 p.m. she never had a problem dropping quickly into sleep. I responded with obvious curiosity to this fact, not knowing what it could mean. Noticing my avid interest, Mildred also volunteered that she likewise had no problem getting to sleep if she waited until after 11 p.m. If she did succeed in getting to sleep between nine and eleven, her night's sleep was inevitably punctuated with restlessness and numerous awakenings. So, here was a curious pattern of great difficulty going to sleep only if she went to bed between nine and eleven p.m. I had never encountered such a pattern and could not identify any rational explanation.

With no logical explanation and uncertain about my next move, I elected to use guided imagery. We obviously needed further information. With Mildred's consent, I led her through a three or four minute abbreviated relaxation exercise while seated in a chair. Once she was breathing slowly and appeared very relaxed with her eyes closed, I asked her to imagine herself suspended on a low hanging cloud above her home. After she nodded in response to my question "Can you see your home clearly?" I suggested that she magically look down into the living quarters of her home at 8:45 p.m. and describe what was happening. Still with eyes closed, she described reading stories of interest in the afternoon newspaper while her husband was finishing drying the supper dishes.

I then asked her to advance the clock to nine p.m. and describe what she saw. Instantly she sucked in a huge breath with a loud audible shriek. "Mildred, tell me what's happening," I said. In a panicky voice she sobbed that the scene had shifted to her childhood home and that her older brother was coming her bedroom. She began sobbing, wailing loudly at this turn of events as she described her brother Jack forcing his sexual attentions on her, beginning when she was twelve years old. I gently terminated the imagery, asked her to open her eyes, and talked with her for some considerable time as she gradually calmed herself from this unexpected insight. The scene had triggered the recall of a series of sexual assaults by her brother which had extended across the greater part of three years. Her mother had blithely dismissed Mildred's futile attempts to find an adult to intervene.

After weeks of intensive therapy, Mildred was able to deal with this tragic episode in her life which foreshadowed many of her future relationship problems with her husband and family. Her psychological work gradually established for herself a better self-image. The key piece of psychological work which enabled her to put the sexual abuse issue behind her and come to a resolution was quintessential and I will describe it here.

This is a process adapted from a very important teacher of mine, Dr. Edith Stauffer (1909-2004) as described in her book *Unconditional Love and Forgiveness*.[27] The five steps that follow describe how I used it with Mildred.

Step one consisted of recognizing and claiming ownership of the demand that Mildred was holding on her brother. Through a cascade of tears, she screamed "He *should* not have done that to me," and "Mother *should* have listened to me and believed me."

Next, after considerable encouragement, Mildred expressed in a loud voice the intense feelings that tumbled out as she recalled the repeated sexual assaults. She expressed her rage at her brother Jack—"I was so mad that I could have killed him," and her own despair—"I was so mortified and emotionally destroyed when he did that to me."

In the third step, I asked her to let herself become aware that maintaining the demands that her brother should not have done this to her would never change him or change what took place. After some time, she was able to understand that hanging on to the demand was only placing herself under continual stress, leading to increased tension, and, in turn, increased physical, emotional and mental distress and illness.

I challenged her: "Since maintaining the demand on Jack doesn't change him one bit, and since maintaining the demand is tending to make you ill, are you ready, then, in your own self interest, to cancel the demand that Jack should not have done this?" With her assent, I then said, "Imagine that Jack is here, sitting on the chair opposite you. He can't say a thing, because he is only imaginary. Tell Jack 'I cancel my demand that you should not have devastated me by raping me. What you did is not o.k., but in my own self-interest, I cancel my demand so that I can let it go'."

In step five, it was essential that Mildred symbolically hand to the imagined brother the responsibility for what he did. I asked her to imagine that she was handing him a tray while saying "Jack, I hand you all the moral, ethical, and cosmic responsibility for what you did; and I wish you well in handling the responsibility from the highest awareness that you know; the total responsibility is now yours."

The act of canceling all the demands was incredibly liberating for her. This is the act of forgiveness which takes place wholly within the mind of the holder of the demand—the "should,"—requiring no necessary contact whatsoever with the perpetrator of the devastating actions. This act of forgiveness tends to re-establish positive attitudes, and immediately reduces the load of stress being carried by the owner of the demand.

As Mildred completed this imaginary dialogue, I could see her shoulders relax, and lines of strain disappear from her face. She began to talk more slowly, and for the first time initiated good eye contact. Mildred broke through the repression of her memory of the event, and absorbed the great feeling of relief and relaxation once she completed the forgiveness exercise. Her anxiety and depression began to ease.

One key to healing may be found already existing in mindful awareness that programs the brain. In some situations, the act of forgiving may be the only path to reducing the stress with which we have been living. The wholly unexpected spontaneous turn in Mildred's guided imagery[41] taught me that sometimes the best thing that I could do as physician or therapist was get out of the way.

Section Ten:
Cancer

Story 34: Ovarian Cancer and Faith

A 67-year-old woman came to my office for a first visit in the spring of 1985. "Helen B." was self-employed as a hairdresser, managing her beauty salon with her husband. Shortly after her first visit, she returned for a periodic physical examination. She was moderately overweight but her heart, lungs, and blood pressure were all quite normal. I did, however, feel something vaguely abnormal in her vagina as if there were a mass present. Though she had previously had a "total" hysterectomy, it was as if part of her cervix had been left behind, or that excessive scar tissue had developed after her surgery. Her routine blood tests indicated compromised liver function and moderate anemia.

I referred her to a gynecologist, but Helen procrastinated, persuaded that her previous physician had described these same abnormal findings several years before. Valuable time was lost trying to locate her previous medical records. Both of her past doctors had retired and her records could not be located. I re-examined her six weeks later and the mass was then distinct and significantly larger.

Her liver function tests were even worse. I viewed all these results as ominous evidence for probable cancer with likely metastatic spread to her liver. With all my persuasive power I became very insistent that she follow advice. She finally agreed to an ultrasound and a liver scan and then a visit to a gynecologist "if the tests show something." She postponed the studies, but relented and visited the gynecologist who found a "mobile mass" which he estimated as "4¾ x 6 inches in size." Kidney and bowel x-rays suggested a "displacing mass" —i.e. cancer. Ultrasound confirmed a "mass in the left pelvis consistent with ovarian origin."

The gynecologist said in his note to me

"I spoke to them—Mrs. [B] and her husband— concerning the risks of this being a malignancy . . . [she] is a very nice lady and appears to be strong willed. She is convinced that this is a benign process . . . She prefers to wait on the surgery until three weeks or so have passed because of her commitment to the new owner of the beauty salon she and her husband have just sold and for whom she is still working. I advised her [that] the longer she delays, the less likely she could be cured with surgery alone."

It still took a month before she finally came to surgery, at which I assisted. A large cancerous mass was present in the left pelvis, extensively involving the small and large bowel. Over 100 1/8 to 3/8 inch-sized masses were scattered throughout the pelvic and abdominal cavities. Five were biopsied. The surgeon's postoperative report described a "Large pelvic mass and possible ovarian carcinoma with tumor encroachment on small bowel involving the lower 2 to 2 1/2 feet as well as tumor involvement of the outside surface of [the] descending colon; [metastatic] peritoneal studding of the surface of small bowel and pelvis." The pathology report of the biopsies revealed:

"Malignant tumor appearing as a poorly differentiated carcinoma, possibly of ovarian origin."

Her ovarian cancer had invaded the large and small bowel, and had spread tiny metastatic cancers all the way up to her liver.

Definitive surgery was postponed for five days to allow for cleansing of the bowel. Removal of the cancer was then undertaken by a general surgeon. A large pelvic cancerous mass 8 ¾ x 7 x 3 inches was removed along with a 39-inch length of small bowel and an 11-inch segment of large bowel. She was left with a colostomy and a remaining rectal bowel segment, with gross amounts of cancer remaining behind. The pathologist described:

"A large mass, terminal ileum and sigmoid colon: poorly differentiated carcinoma [cancer], of probable ovarian origin."

The surgeon's summary recommended ". . . commencement of chemotherapy. The colostomy need not be considered permanent and after chemotherapy, probably within six months, we . . . could close the colostomy."

After recovery from surgery, Helen returned to my office, *protesting her referral* to an oncologist. To my astonishment, she unabashedly said to me *"I want you to tell me what to do to get well!"* I reinforced the necessity for a visit to the oncologist, knowing full well that she would refuse any treatment. I felt professionally uneasy about her choices outside accepted conventional expectations if she did not complete that visit.

Nevertheless, I discussed with her a program, including:

- A low-fat, low-sugar, high fiber diet with ample fruits and vegetables; elimination of red meat and shifting to an intake of all grains in whole, unrefined form.
- Supplementation with large doses of multiple nutritional supplements (see bulleted list below).
- Regular aerobic physical exercise. Since swimming was her only feasible possibility, this was postponed until definitive closing of the colostomy.
- Modifying her attitude toward her husband whom she perceived as critical and controlling, including forgiving and canceling her demands on him.
- Regular meditation, incorporating 1) images of shrinkage and disappearance of the remaining cancer; 2) picturing a hyperactive immune system with scavenger cells destroying all the cancer cells; and 3) imagining and feeling herself totally well and recovered. In her presence, I made an audiotape for her, beginning with a standard relaxation routine followed by the imagery.

Helen's daily supplement schedule:

- 100,000 IU/day of mixed carotenes
- vitamin C increased gradually to 12,000 mg/day
- a megadose multivitamin-multimineral:
    - ~ vitamin E 600 IU
    - ~ selenium 200 mcg
    - ~ calcium 300 mg
    - ~ magnesium 300 mg
    - ~ manganese 6 mg
    - ~ zinc 15 mg
    - ~ copper 1.5 mg
    - ~ 100 mg each of B1, B2, B3 and B6
    - ~ folic acid 800 mcg
    - ~ vitamin B12 400 mcg

On my stern insistence, she relented and did see the oncologist. In his note to me, he stated

" . . . Some of this tumor certainly remains. Mrs. [B], however, *is convinced that she has no residual cancer that requires treatment, or that any residual she does have will be cured by her own body with God's help.* She puts great weight on your opinion and said she would discuss any treatment with you. I made clear my concern that she has residual cancer and that the time to treat would be now rather than later when the tumor is bulkier and chances for a good outcome are much less. Her treatment clearly would not be without side effects and she's aware of that, and this, too, makes her reluctant to undergo any therapy now when she's feeling better from the surgery. I did recommend chemotherapy now rather than later. She's refused for the moment, but is going to discuss this with you. In the meantime I'm going to get [an] abdominal CT scan and tumor marker studies to see if there is any gross residual disease elsewhere." [italics added]

Predictably, Helen B. declined the scan, the tumor marker studies and chemotherapy. Nevertheless, *her blood tests began to steadily improve* and within a month after the original surgeries she was no longer anemic and all her liver function tests were normal. She began to look stronger and exuded confidence that she and God were winning the battle. Her belief in the divine was indomitable and I reinforced her hope with every encouragement.

Her surgeon was unwilling to undertake closure of the colostomy until she had undergone the recommended chemotherapy. She hated the colostomy and pestered the surgeon so persistently that he finally relented, and two and one-half months after her major cancer surgery she was again in surgery, this time to close the colostomy, reconnecting the two parts of the bowel.

The surgery was long and tedious. The adhesions and scar tissue encountered entering the abdominal cavity were among the worst I had ever seen. The hundreds of 1/8 – 3/8 inch peritoneal tumors were present as before and seven of them from various locations were biopsied. With considerable difficulty, the large bowel was reconnected to the rectum. On her third post-operative day the pathology report on the seven biopsies of the small tumors appeared in the chart and described: "Inflammatory tissue with moderate cell variation." *There were no cancer cells in the biopsied tissue!* The surgeon's only unemotional comment about the report, expressed in his Austrian accent was "Vell, she is a vaarry interesting lady."

Helen recovered rapidly from this third surgery. She delighted in her return to normal bowel function and her positive laboratory reports. "I knew they would be o.k.," she said. She returned to the beauty salon and continued to be gainfully employed. She delighted in regular attendance at the Seattle Opera. She traveled to Milan, Italy, to revel in the best opera offered on the European continent. She read Dr. Bernie Siegel's book *Love, Medicine and Miracles* and participated from the audience at a television appearance in Seattle with Dr. Siegel. She had persuaded her husband to build an outdoor Japanese garden in which she continued her daily meditations.

The marital situation with her husband gradually deteriorated, however, in part because he objected to her refusal to undergo conventional treatment. She initiated divorce proceedings about two years after her third surgical procedure. My sense was that this relieved a considerable stress in her life.

In 1987, about three years following her major surgeries, she developed a large, problematic abdominal hernia at the site of the previous operations. She underwent yet a fourth surgery, this time to repair the hernia. At the operation, the surgeon, with my assistance, took advantage of the opportunity to re-explore her abdomen. The scar tissue was totally gone; *there were no residual peritoneal tumors and no evidence of cancer anywhere.*

Following this re-exploration I attempted to get Helen's case scheduled for my hospital's monthly Tumor Board review. I viewed her recovery as an amazing achievement which I thought would interest many of our local doctors. The oncologist chairman, however, on finding that she had not had any definitive conventional treatment beyond surgery, refused to place her on the discussion schedule, saying "If she didn't have any additional treatment, we couldn't learn anything from her case."

In the ensuing five years of her life, she exhibited no evidence of any recurrence of the ovarian cancer. She died at age 75 of totally unrelated causes—complications of an osteoporotic fracture—eight years after her original diagnosis of metastatic cancer.

Did she demonstrate "spontaneous regression" of cancer? Did her immune system respond to the images, the change in attitude, the nutritional initiatives, the ardent hope and belief in divine healing? I do not know what elements in her response to the cancer made the difference, but I was struck by the incontrovertible evidence of complete healing. With her recovery from widespread metastatic cancer I learned a profound lesson: metastatic cancer can sometimes "spontaneously" disappear in a spectacular fashion.

The number of persons who recover from cancer unexpectedly against rational prognostic predictions is probably much larger than we realize. In 1993, the Institute of Noetic Sciences published a summary of over 3,000 documented cases of "spontaneous remission." Caryle Hirshberg and the late Brendan O'Regan scoured decades of medical literature to find these published reports of unexpected recovery from cancer and life-threatening diseases.[40] And from thousands of claims of cures from pilgrims to Lourdes, France, the Roman Catholic Church has authenticated and validated some sixty proven cases for which there is unequivocal medical evidence for cure.[41] These validated reports likely catalogue only a fraction of the instances of healing from cancer. It is very difficult in the conventional medical world to persuade skeptical editors of medical journals to publish documented, proven cases of "spontaneous recovery" from cancer.

The key elements in these healings are difficult to discern and sometimes even unknown, making it problematic to extrapolate what should be imparted to cancer patients to enhance their healing. We do not know enough about 'spontaneous remission' to systematize specific treatment protocols. It may be sufficient for cancer patients to know about these valid healing reports to be able to inject the benefit of hope into their own program for treatment of their disease. I believe we will learn more in the decades to come about how these healings occur.

Story 35: Dave's Metastatic Skin Cancer

Dave, at age 59, appears fit and vigorous. His serious look is interrupted frequently by a broad smile and hearty laugh. As he tells his story, he says it has not always been this way.

When he was 44, he and his wife noticed some changes in a birthmark located over the right lower lumbar region of his back. The lesion was easily irritated, perhaps aggravated by his tool belt which rested across the birthmark. His wife urged him to have it checked. She pushed and nagged, to no avail. Perhaps in denial, Dave resisted going to see a doctor until about four years later, when he noticed an accelerated change in darkening of the birthmark. Simultaneously he noticed the development of a 3/4-inch-sized lump in his right groin. He sought an appointment with a doctor. The birthmark and the lump were excised completely although Dave had expected the doctor would perform a needle biopsy.

Two days later, a second lump appeared in the right groin the size of a walnut. Within days, his physician summarily informed him that the diagnosis was an aggressive stage 2 malignant melanoma which had spread to the lymph glands in his right groin and carried a "77 percent prognosis of dying within five years." His doctor told him he would need additional treatment with chemotherapy. Because of devastating results of chemotherapy in his family members, Dave quickly rejected this recommendation and packed his bags for a visit to the Contreras Clinic in Tijuana, Mexico.

Dave had a strong family history of cancer. His younger brother died at the age of four after developing a rare cancer originating from within the ear. His mother had developed ovarian cancer treated with surgery; she later had breast cancer treated with chemotherapy, after which her cancer metastasized to the lungs. Following lung surgery, she suffered a blood clot in the lung and died. His maternal grandmother had died of cancer. His father developed and recovered from prostate cancer after working for many years with caustic chemicals in an industrial plant. His father-in-law developed cancer of the lung and was told that he had six months to live. Instead he decided to seek treatment at the Contreras clinic in Mexico. Although he survived for fifteen years, he developed a colon cancer after a series of stresses which Dave thinks were related to his cancer. Following his colon cancer, his father-in-law had a recurrence of his lung cancer which progressed to take his life in spite of aggressive conventional treatment. These experiences of his relatives' unsuccessful conventional treatment with their cancers drew Dave to visit the Contreras Clinic in Mexico, where his father-in-law had gone for his successful care resulting in his extended survival.

Dave's early family experiences scripted him to be a high achiever. He worked regularly during college. He was married while in college and his workaholic nature was reinforced by his father-in-law who was a contractor. Dave went to school, worked in the college food service, maintained a marriage, and began working in the home remodeling business. He had fallen into a rather typical American go-go lifestyle at a whirlwind pace.

Prior to the development of his malignant melanoma, Dave's lifestyle was, as he puts it, "free-wheeling." He enjoyed smoking a pipe regularly. He and marijuana were well acquainted. He drank regularly, favoring brandy. He stoked his hunger with fast foods, and a "diet of steak, beer, sugar and white bread." During the time of the gradual changes in his birthmark, he was undergoing tremendous stress as a large-volume builder of spec houses, completing up to 50 in a single year. With a downturn in the housing market, he went deeply into debt to avoid losing everything, carrying at one point fourteen unsold houses on the market, and completely draining a sizable inheritance from his mother to keep his operation from going under.

When Dave arrived at the Contreras Clinic in Tijuana, his operative site in the right groin had become infected and had to be surgically drained. He stopped smoking. He embarked on an educational and treatment program by embracing only the foods offered—an essentially vegetarian diet, fortified with freshly prepared organic fruit and vegetable juices and large amounts of barley grass. He was given supplements of vitamin C, niacin, and amino acids. In his three-week stay, he received regular injections as part of the Alivazantos cancer treatment protocol named for its creator, a well-known Greek physician. The nature of the injections was not divulged to him, but blood tests for cancer markers were done regularly and began to improve. During his three-week sojourn in Mexico, he began to feel stronger, more vigorous, and hopeful. This hope grew rapidly, partly as a result of conversations with returning patients who were doing much better than predicted despite their advanced cancer and poor prognosis.

Dave finally returned to his home in the state of Washington. He read extensively, including descriptions of hydrogen peroxide therapy. He began taking hydrogen peroxide orally three times a day. Far outside the box, the peroxide regime is recommended by a very small group of unconventional doctors. As he embarked on this self-directed, unconventional treatment, he noticed for the first time that his walnut-sized, cancerous lymph node in his right groin began to shrink. He read *Killing Cancer* by Jason Winters. Dave continued drinking large amounts of freshly squeezed and blended vegetable and fruit juices, a routine recommended by a dedicated group of alternative physicians. Dave spent more time in nature, fishing in his favorite streams, hunting chukar (in the pheasant family), and hiking with his dogs on remote trails in the foothills and Cascade Mountains.

Dave also mastered a shift in attitude. He had previously been angry with himself for getting into financial and business problems, not being more successful, and not managing his life better. He decided to forgive himself, and acknowledge and express gratitude for being alive. "I learned to be happy with what I've got." His anger at the world in general gradually subsided and he began to slow down and take life a day at a time. He pictured in his mind the "best ten days of my life," and deliberately began reconnecting often with the activities and the elements in those images. Exploring nature was high on his list.

Family involvement was an integral part of his success. His wife's support of his fresh, whole, organically-grown-foods diet was essential, including adopting it for herself. Her encouragement and support in assisting him in combining all his chosen initiatives also contributed to his positive outlook. He helped to minimize his stress by returning to constructing houses and condominiums on a greatly reduced scale, doing most of the work himself and engaging subcontractors for special parts of the construction process. Some stress remained as his two children left the family nest and were only intermittently employed. He greatly reduced his use of alcohol and marijuana.

Dave discovered that the groin tumor grew when he stopped the hydrogen peroxide. He made contact with a naturopathic physician whose care was completely consistent with his chosen direction. He began to prepare and consume Essiac tea, on one occasion going on a 60-mile hike and drinking large amounts of this tea—during which time his tumor noticeably regressed. Following this, he greatly increased his walking.

He embarked on a trial of intravenous vitamin C treatments from his physician. After his first intravenous infusion of 50 grams of vitamin C he felt impressively energized and "fired up" for two weeks. He continued to receive one to two vitamin C infusions a week[42,43,44] for many months, and added long hydrogen peroxide soaks in the tub.

From the time of his cancer diagnosis at age 48, his walnut-sized lymph node in his groin provided him with a marker for the progress of his self-designed treatment. A steady shrinkage occurred over a four-year period, interrupted by periods of temporary enlargement whenever he relaxed his successful dietary and treatment options. Gradually, his tumor shrank to the size of an almond, then finally shriveled to such a tiny size it could no longer be felt. Accompanying this was a global sense of greater vigor, energy, positivity, and enthusiasm. I first met Dave as I co-facilitated a support group for cancer patients, where he continued to learn and add to the changes in lifestyle which he intuitively sensed were helpful.

Is Dave cured? A scientific answer would be "no one knows." Oncologists frequently talk in terms of "five-year-cures." Dave at this writing has survived fifteen years from the time his birthmark began to change. With completely normal blood chemistry profiles and physical examinations, a reasonable conclusion would be that he is recovered. Dave does not say that. He is very certain, however, that the cancer is under control. And beyond that, he looks and feels better and consciously acknowledges appreciation for every day of life he has been given. In 2011, Dave continues to do well with no signs of recurrence.

Dave's experience taught me that there are many factors involved in recovery from metastatic cancer—nutrition, exercise, attitude, and beliefs. And specific treatments, even those outside the accepted norms of conventional medicine, appear to be valuable for specific people with specific cancers. Dave tried many things, and benefited from having a marker (the palpable lymph node) to give him feedback about which things were helping. Dave thinks that relief from stress and a marked shift in lifestyle were big factors in his recovery.

My view of cancer and its treatment expanded as I observed Dave steadily improve over the years of his self-selected treatments. The vast majority of patients diagnosed with cancer undergo treatment with the conventional medical approach of surgery, chemotherapy, and radiation. Although the "cause" of cancer is usually described as unknown, there is an important lesson in the realization that cancer is almost unknown in the few remaining indigenous primitive tribes of the world. And cancer was known, but rare, in "advanced" societies until the early 1800s during the industrial revolution. These statistics can be validated even after allowing for the shorter lifespan of indigenous tribal members and pre-industrial revolution peoples.

Dave's remarkable recovery with unconventional treatment involving no chemotherapy or radiation forced me to think more broadly about the effectiveness of different therapies to cancer. Conventional treatment of cancer can also result in long-term remissions and cures in many instances. We will make progress in this arena only when we openly evaluate each offered cancer treatment without preconceived prejudices. Treatment for cancer and every human malady must be individualized and must consider every known variable from patient to patient. A single uniform approach does not work for everyone.

Story 36: Kenneth's Stress and His Cancer

I had been the family doctor for Kenneth, age 41, his wife, Karen, a registered nurse, and their three girls. I had seen Kenneth infrequently, however, and never for anything major. He had not taken the time for a complete physical examination, and indeed it took considerable urging by his wife to see a doctor at all. When I did see him, he seemed introverted, didn't talk much, and manifested a flattened emotional expression as if depression might be lurking beneath the surface.

At his appointment, he removed his shirt and revealed an ugly-looking skin tumor about 2/3 of the size of a dime on the right upper chest. He had noticed it about a month before and thought that it had grown. It was slightly raised, and faintly reddish-purple. Because of its ominous appearance as a malignant melanoma, I took the time during that appointment to remove it with a generous surgical margin.

As I was injecting the local anesthetic and performing the excision, Kenneth talked about what was going on in his life. He had lost his sales job about 15 months before when the company for which he worked was acquired by another firm. He described his loss of self-esteem, and feelings of shame and worthlessness as his family went through a financial crisis. He felt badly about becoming totally dependent on his wife's income, and exhausting much of their savings. As he repeatedly failed to land another job, self-loathing mounted, overlain with anxiety over the likelihood of having to take a significant cut in pay to work at all.

The pathology report returned three days later and confirmed that the tumor was a "Clark's Level 3 malignant melanoma with aggressive characteristics." This classification meant his cancer was rated a three on a scale of four for severity. His wound healed well and there was no evidence that the tumor had spread into the regional lymph glands in the armpit or beyond. As I removed his sutures ten days later, I was struck by his bright demeanor and his upbeat conversation. He had found a new job in the meantime and was scheduled to start work the following Monday. I did suggest that he consult an oncologist, and later confirmed that he had declined in spite of his wife's urging.

Kenneth, however, remained well and over the years showed no signs of recurrence of his melanoma. I rarely saw him, but on numerous occasions inquired of his status on seeing his wife and children in my office.

To my surprise, nearly ten years later, he came to the office with two hard lymph nodes in his right armpit. On biopsy they proved to be a recurrence of his malignant melanoma. I learned that about fifteen months before this cancer recurrence, he had lost the job which he had secured at the time of the original surgery. He again appeared morose, withdrawn, defeated, and depressed. His description of the recent recurrence was very difficult for him to express. He had discovered the lumps four months before and had done nothing about them. He refused all treatment, and died quickly about four months later.

I had to ask myself, "What was the malignant melanoma doing for nearly ten years?" I had to logically assume that, following the original surgery, there must have been residual cancer in the tissues. I could only conclude that his immune system had held the cancer at bay for over nine years while he was earning a living and felt happy and relatively good about himself. With the loss of his job since I saw him last, hopelessness and helplessness had again set in, causing his immune defenses to be compromised by the stress of being unemployed.

Kenneth's experience highlighted for me the relationship of stress and depression to the onset of disease including cancer and cancer recurrence. His story prompted me to pay much greater attention to the presence of stress in the lives of my patients, acknowledge it, and take steps to help them neutralize its devastating effects.

Commonly held opinions in medical cancer literature still hold that stress is an unproven factor in cancer or its recurrence. Kenneth's story, however, with his death at age 51, told me that in some instances, the influence of stress is a major factor. Perhaps the best confirmation for the relationship of stress to the onset of threatening illness comes from the recognized increase in several degenerative diseases, including cancer, in elderly surviving widows and widowers. Compared to those whose spouses are living, the death rate of widows and widowers is significantly greater during the 18-month window of time following the death of the spouse.

The timing of Kenneth's stressful job losses to the original appearance and later the recurrence of his malignant melanoma seems too obvious to ignore. In retrospect I had some regret for not making the connection more quickly and helping him address the issues underlying his stress. The lesson may be for all of us to pay attention to the impact of stress in our own lives and take steps to neutralize its effects. Medical evidence now clearly demonstrates that most persons can, with or without professional help, greatly limit the toxic effects of stress.

Section Eleven:
What's The Source Of Healing?

Story 37: Healing Outside the Norm

Malcolm and his family had been patients in my family practice for several years. In his early forties, Malcolm stood six-feet two with an athletic build and an engaging personality. He worked in a successful local business in which he had some partial financial interest and management role. He always struck me as the essential example of a young "pillar of society:" strong family relationships, successful business career, participant in his church and community affairs, athletic interests, and health consciousness. He was the essence of my primary care physician's example of what I would hope all patients would be like.

On a late Saturday afternoon in the early fall I received a message from Malcolm through my answering service. On returning the call, I learned from a family member that Malcolm had injured his right knee while water skiing on a lake about 25 miles from our community. Emergency Medical Technicians on the scene had placed his leg in a cardboard splint and sent him off to our local hospital in the back seat of his car. The family had stopped by their residence and placed the call to my answering service because he wanted to be seen at my office rather than going to our hospital emergency room. With some hesitation I consented to see him, but warned them that we might need access to x-rays at the hospital.

About 45 minutes later, he hobbled into the office on borrowed crutches. I knew from prior experience that he had a high pain tolerance, but his body language gave me the impression of severe discomfort. Gingerly removing the cardboard splint, I examined his knee. There was surprisingly little swelling for the twisting injury he sustained as he tumbled off his water ski. There was marked tenderness over the inside of his right knee. Carefully bending his knee, physical testing for intactness of the internal cruciate ligaments of the knee was normal. On carefully checking his knee in the straightened position to ascertain the intactness of the major medial collateral ligament on the inside of the knee, I succumbed to a sinking feeling as I met *no resistance at all* in springing his knee apart. The major ligament on the inside of the knee which holds the knee joint together had been completely torn off its attachment to the tibial bone of the lower leg.

Placing his right leg carefully back in the splint, I told him that it would be necessary to undergo surgery to reattach the torn lower end of the medial collateral ligament to the tibia. I was prepared to go on and talk about referral to an orthopedic surgeon when he asked, "What would happen if we let it heal on its own?"

Aghast, I told him politely that this was an irrational and very risky choice; in all likelihood the ligament would not reattach itself to the tibia, and that if it did, it would likely heal in such a way as to make the knee permanently unstable. The more we talked, the more Malcolm became insistent on embarking on this conservative treatment without surgery. After a few minutes, I knew that he was not going to consent to a surgical repair.

I asked him to sign a disclaimer in his chart that he was knowingly rejecting the recommended surgical treatment and would accept the consequences of his choice. His wife, who was present throughout the visit, was also dubious about his choice, but we were forced to accept it.

I placed the leg in a long-leg plaster cast to prevent motion in the knee, gave him a prescription for a few moderately strong pain pills (which he never filled), and made an appointment for him to be seen in four days. At that visit, *he had returned to work,* experiencing pain that was tolerable, and expressing great confidence that the knee would heal. In the meantime I had talked with my orthopedic surgeon, who thought he undoubtedly faced a terrible result with severe malfunction of the knee.

For six weeks, we repaired the plaster cast as it cracked and disintegrated. Removing it for the final time, I kept the knee firmly wrapped, and asked him to begin cautious motion. He rejected my suggestion to work with a physical therapist in the rehabilitation process, preferring to work on his rehab by himself. As the weeks passed, he gradually increased his activity. Successive checks of the knee showed that the *ligamentous deficit was healing and the knee exam showed progressive tightening* as I checked for resistance by attempting to spring the knee apart. I was incredulous at the healing of the ligament to its proper attachment on its own schedule without the benefit of surgery. Malcolm seemed totally accepting of this result, and did not even say "I told you so."

Malcolm returned to water skiing the following summer without a problem and with a fully functioning knee. Two years later he tore the same ligament *again*, once more refusing surgical treatment. All of us at the office watched as his knee again healed "on its own."

Malcolm's quiet confidence was grounded in great trust in his own healing capacity as well as a strong religious faith which I sensed somehow contributed to his healing. He was more cautious about water skiing after the second incident, but remained athletically active in strenuous activities including hiking in the Cascade Mountains of our state.

This was, of course, a shocking surprise to me to observe a complete recovery of a severely injured, critical structure of Malcolm's body totally outside the guidelines of standard medical practice. I now believe there is embedded in our human experience a potential for the physical body, and perhaps the mental and emotional bodies as well, to heal themselves. While not recommending Malcolm's choice to others, I learned that it is important that we do nothing to interfere with the inner healing potential.

Story 38: A clinical revelation
(while standing barefoot in an inch
of water in the San Francisco Airport)

In the mid-1960s, I become acquainted with a family in my community who later sought my medical care for their children. One of their three offspring was a bright teenager who began to progressively gain weight while in high school. Andrew had a stocky build, resembling his father who also had a large frame. He participated in sports but his weight progressively crept upward to the point they sought medical help.

On his first office visit, Andrew appeared to be about fifty to sixty pounds overweight. I asked a flock of questions, including those related to his nutritional history. It seemed that Andrew was not overeating. He talked of being easily fatigued and complained that his skin was dry. His tendon reflexes were sluggish. These clues led me to obtain blood for a complete blood count, serum chemistries and thyroid tests. Sure enough, his tests returned a verdict of a low thyroid hormone level (hypothyroidism).

I prescribed one grain of natural thyroid daily. I had by this time found that for many (but not all) hypothyroid patients, "natural" thyroid derived from the whole thyroid glands of animals worked better than laboratory-manufactured synthetic thyroid hormone. Over several months, increased doses of thyroid guided by his clinical improvement and repeated testing began to change his metabolism, and he progressively lost weight. On three grains of thyroid daily (180 mg) his weight leveled out at near ideal, his fatigue was completely gone, and his thyroid function tests came into the normal range.

The next year he left home to attend college in California. I continued to see his siblings, but heard nothing from the family about Andrew's thyroid condition.

About ten years later, I was returning from making a presentation at a Bay Area Family Practice Residency Consortium retreat near Monterrey, California. Following the retreat, I returned to the San Francisco airport in my rental car, arriving in the midst of a driving rainstorm. My flight was scheduled to leave from a concourse which was being reconstructed. The jetways were not yet functioning and I was scheduled to board my flight by means of a stairway from the level of the tarmac. I was warned on checking in that the waiting areas on the ground level of my concourse were flooded by the rainstorm. On descending the escalator, I could see hundreds of people waiting for flights while sloshing around in water over an inch deep, shoes and socks in hand. I found the scene quite comical with strangers animatedly talking with each other about the very unusual conditions.

Suddenly I heard someone say "Dr. Anderson!" I turned to see Andrew, standing in bare feet along with everyone else. I did not immediately recognize him. "I'm Andrew," he said. On matching his name to my recollection I greeted him warmly and we fell to talking for about twenty minutes before I heard the boarding call for my flight. I was eager to hear about what had transpired in his life since leaving home after high school.

After a year or two of college, he had become motivated to switch to a Bible college in California. He had received his undergraduate degree but did not enter the ministry, electing instead to earn his living in the business world. I was curious about his thyroid condition, and he related his story.

After being in college in California for about a year he had begun to lose weight. He sought care at the campus health center where he was seen by a doctor who retested him for his thyroid function and found that he was taking too much thyroid supplement and reduced his dosage. Over a period of several months, his dose of thyroid was progressively decreased to the point he was finally taken off thyroid completely. It was then that he realized that the weight loss, signaling a thyroid overdosage, had started very quickly *after he had undergone an abrupt religious conversion.* His conversion markedly shifted his worldview and was the chief factor in deciding to shift his education to a Bible college. His conversion had suddenly changed his metabolism in such a way that he no longer needed any thyroid supplement medication.

This story did not conform itself to the principles of medicine

I had learned in my training. I have not experienced this healing phenomenon related to a religious conversion in any other patient. I could only express my joy at the fact that his thyroid condition had been healed. My belief system shifted again.

Many of these stories hint at the fact that human beings, and perhaps most life species, have a capacity for self-healing. The previous story of the healing of Malcolm's knee injury (Story 37) is testimony to that capacity. For many, faith in a divine providence is one of the threads interwoven with many other strands of healing to create our tapestry of health.

Section Twelve:
Mysterium

Story 39: The Disappearing Pediatrician

Our first grandchild, a six pound nine-ounce girl, was born in the early 1990s after a full-term pregnancy. Our son, a navy SEAL, called us about 7 a.m. from the hospital in Novato, California, north of San Francisco, to tell us the good news. The labor had been about 11 hours and the birth APGAR score was a 9 (a score of 9 or 10 indicates a healthy birth condition). The hospital had assigned a pediatrician to her case. My son described him as a short, very slender man with rugged features, a unique bearing and a pronounced limp from what appeared to be a shortened leg. He performed the routine newborn examination of our granddaughter shortly before my son's call, finding her healthy with all systems functioning normally. He exhibited a professional but pleasant demeanor as he stopped to talk with our son and his wife to answer their questions.

To the surprise of our son and daughter-in-law, the pediatrician reappeared at the hospital about 11 a.m. to recheck our granddaughter. While he was re-examining her, our son talked with the nurses, who said that they had not noticed any problem and *had not called the pediatrician.* On completing his examination, the pediatrician asked them to sign permission to perform a lumbar puncture to check for meningitis. Our son had enough medical knowledge to realize this meant there was a potentially alarming problem. With considerable anxiety, they signed the permit and learned soon afterward that the spinal fluid confirmed the suspicion of meningitis.

Our son called us again shortly after noon with the discouraging news. The pediatrician made arrangements to transfer our newborn granddaughter to San Francisco Children's Hospital by ambulance and asked her parents to follow in their car. My son asked the neonatologist, who was assigned to her case at the San Francisco hospital, to call me, particularly because I was a physician. Late that afternoon, I received a call from the very competent neonatologist assigned to our granddaughter's care. She explained our granddaughter's condition and her planned treatment. Over the next week she reached me three more times to apprise me of what was going on.

Newborn meningitis carries a 25 percent risk of brain injury and/or mental retardation, and a significant possibility of death. For three days, three different antibiotics were administered intravenously through 25-gauge needles in her scalp veins until the identification and antibiotic sensitivity of the bacterium were known. The organism turned out to be a type B streptococcus. Our granddaughter responded nicely to the antibiotics and did well with no evidence of any adverse effects on her brain and nervous system. After three weeks, she was discharged to her parents who took her home for the first time.

A week later they had an appointment with the pediatrician who had first checked her in the Novato hospital. All was well. A followup visit after one more week again took place in the pediatrician's office in a medical office building in Novato. They made an appointment to return for a final checkup one month later.

Arriving for that visit, *they found the office suite vacated and no name plate on the door.* Totally perplexed, they asked in an adjacent medical office where the pediatrician had gone. No one in the adjacent office had ever heard of a doctor by that name. Further, the receptionist said "You must be mistaken, that office has been vacant for over six months." A receptionist in another office in the building had likewise never heard of the pediatrician. He was not listed in the yellow pages. The Marin [County] Medical Society had no record of him. Totally baffled, our son and daughter-in-law later took her to another pediatrician recommended by a Navy buddy.

Our son called us a few weeks later about the incident. He is a no-nonsense, tough, Navy SEAL, not given to thinking much about vanishing pediatricians. Nonetheless, responding to my question of what he thought of this mystery, he ventured his thought that *perhaps the doctor had been an angel masquerading as a pediatrician.* Although this stretched my credulity, I was not about to argue, given the early discovery and healthy recovery from the meningitis. I could not venture a rational explanation for either the "disappearing act" or the re-appearance by the pediatrician on the day of our granddaughter's birth when he had not been summoned by the nursery personnel.

The final chapter of this story was recently written. On

requesting the records from the Novato hospital where she was born, copies of two emergency room visits during her first year of life were located; the obstetrician's record of her mother's labor, delivery, and post-partum hospitalization were located; but *the inpatient record of the pediatrician's newborn care of our granddaughter was strangely missing from the archives.*

I do not know how often people experience the unexplainable. When I tell this story and ask how many in an audience have had a mysterious experience, I typically find a show of hands of about 40 percent. But we do not often share these "irrational" experiences for fear of appearing weird. If we pay attention, I believe that we can tune in to events occurring at the margins of reality where mystery still holds sway. This experience stretched my worldview into a zone of radical change.

Had I heard this story from someone else, I would have had difficulty believing it and might have totally discounted it as a fabrication. But when my ultra-rational son and daughter-in-law experienced it, I had to honor it and shift my worldview. Abject skepticism would not allow me to live comfortably with rejection of this valid and mystifying encounter.

Story 40: Wake Up!

It was September of 1965. In July of that year, my wife and I with our two children had moved into a newly built home in our Seattle suburb. We had retired to bed about 9:30 p.m., as the last glow of sunset from behind the Olympic Mountains and Puget Sound gradually gave way to the evening darkness.

We were abruptly awakened at about two a.m. by a thunderous noise which vibrated the entire house. We instantly rolled out of our respective sides of our bed, our attention immediately drawn to a brilliant light outside our undraped windows. About fifteen feet from our second story windows was a sun-like spherical form with swirling colors of yellow, white and orange. I later recalled this image, whatever it was, as about three and one-half feet in diameter. Eruptions on the surface of the phenomenon were coordinated with M-80-like explosive sounds.

My wife and I stared at each other in disbelief. My thoughts in quick succession were: Could this be a dream? Not with two of us experiencing it. Why weren't all the neighbors awakened with the thunderous noise? Is this a UFO? And then came fear. Was this threatening in some way? To my wife I suggested, "I'll check the kids, why don't you check the house?" We raced from the bedroom. I found our two children in their respective bedrooms, fast asleep and oblivious of any problem.

My wife ran the length of the house, and on entering the kitchen became aware of the acrid smell of smoke. Beside the back door at the far end of the kitchen stood the ironing board with the iron placed upright and turned off. She had been ironing before coming to bed. But we had neglected a frayed ironing cord which was just sputtering into flame where it had lain smoldering against the ironing board cover. She unplugged the cord and set the entire ironing board outside the back door, leaving the door ajar.

We arrived back in the bedroom, finding the phenomenon gone. On rechecking the house again, we closed the back door. We sat on the edge of the bed in stunned silence for what seemed like an hour, totally unable to grasp or comprehend what we had just experienced.

The rest of the night we talked, unable to force the experience into the box of rationality. Later, we found that none of the neighbors were aware of any disturbances or noise.

Debunkers of our experience have interpreted the phenomenon as "ball lightning." Ball lightning is a recognized event associated with severe electrical storms in which lightning assumes a spherical ball shape two or three feet off the ground. On this particular September night, the weather was calm for a hundred miles in all directions.

We did not share the experience with anyone for some time, fearing that we might be considered loony and given to hallucinations. It was years before we shared it with our children after they had grown to an age when they could possibly understand to some degree. Again, to us, this felt like a mystical experience from the margins of reality. Others have postulated the intervention of a "protective angel."

I could only say that we had clearly been warned to wake up and that our home was about to catch fire. We expressed gratitude for whatever mysterious force provided the wakeup experience. My worldview shifted dramatically through this experience. It happened, we observed it, we paid attention.

I have often thought of this experience as the ultimate in preventive care.

Story 41: Myrtle Calling

The Dempsey family members had been patients in my family medical practice for several years. The mother, Myrtle, was a registered nurse. The father, Henry, was a psychiatrist who had a busy psychoanalysis practice in a downtown Seattle medical office building. They had four boys, who, at the time of this story, ranged in age from late teenagers to their early twenties. Most of my medical contacts were with Myrtle and the boys. In our suburban community, we were also socially acquainted with the family, working together on civic and hospital projects.

Henry, in his early fifties, had experienced a heart attack three years previously, while he was at work in his office in Seattle. He had been successfully treated by a cardiologist in the hospital near his office, returning to normal activities in about six weeks.

On a Thursday evening, I had retired to bed about nine o'clock in the evening. Before I fell asleep, the telephone rang, and I reached for the phone beside our bed. While lifting the handset from the phone, an instant before being able to answer, I saw in my mind's eye a visual image of the outside of Henry and Myrtle's home as if I were viewing it from the street. I knew that I would be speaking with someone from the Dempsey household.

I had not had any contact with any member of the family for several months. In anxious phrases, Myrtle nervously explained that Henry was having tightness in his chest. She had called his cardiologist, who was out of town. She was referred to another cardiologist on call, who, after some discussion, told her to give Henry two aspirin and call him in the morning. After Myrtle's description, I said "I'm calling the ambulance (this was before the 9-1-1 era) and I'll meet you at the hospital." In the emergency room of our suburban hospital, an electrocardiogram confirmed that he was having another heart attack. He was admitted to the hospital and aided by appropriate treatment by my cardiologist and myself, he successfully recovered.

How do we explain premonitions? Dr. Larry Dossey has written extensively about the mystery of documented premonitory experiences and potential explanations of how they can be perceived (*The Power of Premonitions*, 2007). A theoretical explanation requires stepping outside the realm of conventional science. In time I believe we will eventually have a more complete explanation for this and similar "paranormal" mystical experiences. In the meantime, we can confirm that people do have such experiences more often than we realize.

Many persons experiencing precognitive phenomena have not shared their stories with others, largely for fear of being perceived as weird or strange. It is important to pay attention to these experiences, and test their validity. Just as Copernicus upset the world's assumption of an earth-centered solar system in 1543 on publishing his observation that the earth revolved around the sun, so new experiences and observations will continue to shed new light on the more exact nature of who we are and how we relate to the entire cosmos.

Story 42: Introduction To Intuition

In the early 1980s, one of the families in my primary care medical practice moved to another community about thirty miles away. For quite some time, they continued to return to my office for their medical care in spite of the burden of the distance. I had delivered their young daughter, Cecile, 18 months before.

The parents brought Cecile to the office with a high fever of 104°F. I did a thorough evaluation, unable to identify any of the more common causes of such a high fever. On examining the child and gently flexing her head forward on her chest, my hands met a subtle resistance. This has been described as a "doughy" or sticky feeling. Having over the years examined a number of children with meningitis presenting with this subtle finding, I told the young parents that we needed to do a lumbar puncture ("spinal tap").

An hour later, we gathered in the Emergency Room of our hospital across the street from my office. With the help of a nurse in the ER and the mother holding the child, I injected a local anesthetic to minimize the pain of insertion of the larger needle into the envelope of spinal fluid surrounding Cecile's spinal cord. It was common at that time to ask a parent to hold the child firmly while lying on her/his side with the spine bent forward to facilitate entry of the spinal needle as easily as possible.

A few drops of clear spinal fluid were dripped into a sterile test tube and sent to the lab for analysis. A few minutes later, we learned that all aspects of the test were normal. I breathed a sigh of relief and reassured the parents. I suggested measures to try and keep the fever below 102°F and asked them to call the office with a progress report the next day.

By the next morning, Cecile's temperature continued fluctuating between 102°and 104°F. She was not eating and whimpered with generalized discomfort. We asked the parents to bring her in again in the afternoon for me to reexamine her. There were no new definitive clues. The neck examination again revealed subtle resistance to bending her head forward.

Immediately, before I had time to analyze the situation and

rationally decide what to do, I said, "I hate to tell you this, but we need to do another lumbar puncture." Both parents looked startled, and amazingly enough, murmured, "Well, o.k. if you think so." I later reflected on the trust they must have had to not even question my judgment.

We repeated the procedure; the drops of spinal fluid looked cloudy and the lab reported 300 white cells present in each milliliter of fluid, confirming the diagnosis of meningitis. With appropriate antibiotics, guided by the culture obtained from the second spinal fluid specimen, Cecile recovered quickly with no aftereffects.

Only some years later after my worldview had migrated further outside the conventional box, did I realize that it was my intuition which overrode my logical thinking in suggesting a repeat lumbar puncture. The intuition is not understood well enough to be a consistently reliable source of information available at any time on demand. And we do not well understand the source of intuitive hits when they happen. They are often, however, worth checking out; Cecile's parents thought so.

As I broadened my thinking, I am now aware that being open to the possibility of tuning in to the intuition increases the likelihood of connecting with it, whatever "it" is, in meaningful ways. Was my intuitive outburst irrational? I like to think of it as supra-rational.

Story 43: Lost Papers

Mark, a tall, blond, engaging young man, adapted nicely to the role of medical student while seeing patients in my family medical office. He was in the second year of medical school at the University of Washington School of Medicine in Seattle. As part of his training, he spent one half-day each week with me in my office for a year to learn the principles of clinical history-taking and physical examination. He was a quick study and soon learned to comfortably relate to patients in very positive ways as his fund of medical knowledge grew. Each Thursday morning he rode his motorcycle north from the University district to my office about fourteen miles away.

In the winter quarter he told me that he was working on a research project with one of his instructors at the Medical School. Would I be interested in seeing his paper? Of course I was, and asked him to bring with him the draft of his paper when it was finished.

Two weeks later, he started from his room in the University district with the draft of his paper secured under the spring-loaded clips on the back of his motorcycle. As he walked into the office, my staff knew there was something terribly wrong. He was ashen, anxious, and on the verge of panic. When he arrived at the office and turned to take his manuscript from the clips on the back of the motorcycle, there were only four sheets remaining of his 75-page manuscript. In the 1980s before the era of computers and saved documents, his manuscript had been typewritten with no carbon copies. The four-page index of all his references at the end of his draft was part of the missing papers. Mark was devastated.

Impulsively, I quickly reassured him. "When we finish seeing patients this morning," I said, *"we'll meditate to find out where they are and go find them!"* A second later, my rational self began a drumbeat of doubt. And with dilated pupils Mark stared incredulously at me as if to ask, "Am I studying with a rational doctor?"

After seeing patients together all morning, I asked my staff to hold all calls and we retreated to my office where I led the two of us in a brief relaxation exercise with eyes closed. I followed this with an instruction: "Now in your mind's eye allow a picture of the location of the missing papers to appear." Captured by anxiety, Mark envisioned absolutely no images of value, but quickly, in my own mind's eye, I saw papers scattered along the base of a steep fifty-foot embankment. Startled at this immediate image, I soon terminated the exercise. Mark described for me the route he had taken from the University to my office. As I reviewed the route in my mind, there was only one location which fit the description — along the north-bound lanes of the I-5 freeway, running north and south through Seattle, near the Northgate Shopping Mall.

We drove together to a freeway entrance south of the presumed location. We then entered the freeway traveling northbound. As I drove slowly on the right hand shoulder past the steep embankment, Mark looked intently toward the bottom of the slope on our right. No papers. "I'm sure they're here," I said, again immediately enveloping my confident statement with inner doubt. We got off the freeway, looped south and again entered the northbound lanes, this time hugging the inside shoulder with Mark peering into the wooded median on our left. Suddenly, he shouted elatedly "There's one!" While I drove slowly along the shoulder for the next half-mile, he ran in and out of the trees and shrubbery in the wide median, picking up 67 of the missing 71 sheets of his manuscript, including his four pages of references.

Mark's panic-stricken appearance quickly shifted to one of joyous relief. He struggled to try to fit this cognitive real-time experience into the rational, scientific approach to life he was learning in medical school.

I learned with this encounter to be open to the mysterious experience discussed by twentieth century European psychiatrists Carl Jung and Roberto Assagioli, who described a "collective unconscious." William James, the Psychologist-Philosopher-Physician of a hundred years ago also wrote extensively on the varieties of mystical experiences.

In recent decades, the term "remote viewing" has been used to describe the phenomenon of "seeing" things at a distance. In a project terminated in 1995, the U.S. government investigated these capabilities, probing the possible military advantages of information derived from remote viewing. Many persons have had the experiences of finding that a hunch or intuition turned out to be accurate. In this instance, my image was not wholly accurate, but close enough to lead us to the location of Mark's missing papers across the freeway. Such inexplicable experiences are more likely to happen when we are open to possibilities which move beyond the limitations of accepted, conventional science. There are simply times when we brush against the margins of reality which are intermingled with the mysterious. Whether the experience is rational or mysterious, it is essential to pay attention.

I learned from my experience with Mark that in the broadest sense we are all students in the world of real-time life experience.

Story 44: Silent Communication

William and the members of his family had been patients in my family medicine practice for over a decade. In his 50s, William was an engineer who worked for one of the larger commercial engineering firms in the U.S. His wife had been a stay-at-home mother to their five children while managing to be highly active in many church and community activities.

She called our office on a Thursday, a day and a half before my family and I were due to leave on a two-week late summer vacation. She described her concern at watching her left-handed husband's increasing use of his right arm and hand over several weeks. That morning she had seen him use his right hand to shave with his electric razor. I acknowledged her concern while trying to conceal my deep sense of alarm at the threatening nature of her observations. We hastily arranged to squeeze William into the office schedule the following day on Friday.

On examination, William's balance was mildly compromised and his left arm muscle strength was diminished. Among the diagnoses which quickly filtered through my thinking was "brain tumor." Without mentioning that specifically, I communicated the urgent need to follow up with his serious symptoms. I reached my neurologist consultant, and by using the "you owe me one" argument, I persuaded him to see William the following morning on Saturday. I sent William and his wife off with a handwritten referral note to the neurologist.

On returning home from our vacation two weeks later, I was horrified to learn from William's wife that he had canceled the hastily arranged Saturday visit with the neurologist and had taken no additional steps to see any one else. I reached William on the phone and with all the urgency I could muster, insisted that he follow my recommendations. "Bill, you MUST . . . " Between my coercive language and the passionate demands of his wife, William relented, saw the neurologist and submitted to a battery of tests which showed that he had a brain tumor in a very advanced stage. Based on the available information, the best educated guess was that it was either an astrocytoma or a glioblastoma, very aggressive, and nearly always fatal brain cancers.

The neurosurgeon to whom he was later referred told him his only hope for extending his life lay in surgery to remove as much of the cancer as possible. Surgery was scheduled at a Seattle hospital on a Monday morning. William and his wife were warned that one of the possible outcomes was that he might never awaken from the anesthetic after the operation. The surgery was very difficult, and the cancer more extensive than had been suggested by the tests. It was impossible to remove the greatest bulk of the cancer, leaving William with the probability of surviving only a short time.

Because our suburban community was a 45 minute drive into the city, William's wife had hastily arranged bed and breakfast lodging near the hospital. She visited him several times a day in the intensive care unit at the hospital. William remained unconscious, his life prolonged only by a respirator. Each morning his wife called me at home to apprise me of the situation. Each morning of that week, on arriving at the office, I informed my staff of William's condition.

On Thursday morning she tearfully informed me that William had died during the night at 2:20 a.m., while still on the respirator. I expressed my condolences and asked her to keep me informed about decisions for a memorial service and made myself available to speak with her at any time.

On arriving at the office that morning, before I could inform my staff about William's death, my office nurse described a vivid dream in which she realized that William had died. I asked her if she had been awakened by her dream. "Oh, yes, the dream was so real," she replied. "What time was it?" I asked, avoiding telling her what I already knew. "It was 2:20," she replied.

I then informed everyone that William had, indeed, died at 2:20 a.m. The entire staff, including my nurse, looked astonished and incredulous, unable to rationally understand how the two events had coincided.

How do persons in a dream become aware of what is happening in a remote location twenty miles away? Authorities wiser than I posit a variety of explanations. For me, these occurrences are still thinly veiled events seen through hazy glass at the margins of reality. Perhaps as human experience develops, one day we shall know.

I am certain that people experience these events far more commonly than most realize. We tend to downplay these experiences, live in denial about them, or hide them from others because we think naysayers will belittle us. When more people merely report their experiences, human progress will leap forward.

Afterword

As these forty-four stories crossed the stage of my experience in forty years of primary care medical practice, I was moved step by step to think more broadly outside the limitations of my own education and medical training. My conventional training was of the highest quality I can imagine, but the impact of the events cited in these vignettes kept shifting my worldview as a result of paying attention, observing carefully and thinking reflectively in unlimited ways.

Close observations have forced me to think more and more about the constant state of change taking place in our concepts of becoming ill, living, dying, and seeking cures and healing. Critics may find no merit in some of the stories, several of which are not explained with principles of accepted conventional science. They may simply discount such experiences as fabricated. However, society ignores valid, anomalous experiences to its own detriment.

Austrian physician Ignaz Semmelweis recorded his observations of post-partum infections in the birthing hospitals of Vienna in 1847. When obstetricians followed his admonition to wash their hands between patient examinations, the death rate from infections after childbirth fell from about twelve percent to less then two percent. His success incurred the jealous wrath of his colleagues. He was savagely attacked, vilified, and committed to an insane asylum where he suffered an ignominious death in obscurity in 1865. Then, ten years later, a sculpture of his likeness was raised in Budapest in his honor!

The renowned engineer, Nikola Tesla, born in 1856 in what is now Croatia, began his career as an electrical engineer with a telephone company in Budapest in 1881. While walking with a friend through a city park, the elusive solution to the rotating magnetic field problem flashed through his mind. With a stick, he drew a diagram in the sand, explaining to his friend the principle of the induction motor. This principle became the basis for the now universal generation of alternating current electricity created from falling water and the burning of fossil fuels.

The German chemist Friedrich August Kekulé mused in a

daydream in his laboratory in 1865. Kekulé realized that the chemical reactions of carbon he had been intensely studying for two years could not be explained with then known straight- and branched-carbon-chain formulas. In a quiet moment of reverie, while staring into the dying embers of his fireplace, the rising heat waves appeared to him to turn into writhing snakes, which suddenly, as if by a signal, grasped themselves by their own tails. Within days, Kekulé was able to explain the chemical reactions by realizing that carbon formulas also exist in circles. The secret of the hexagonal benzene ring was unmasked, and biochemistry took an enormous leap forward.

In 1928, Alexander Fleming observed the inhibition of the growth of bacteria in a Petrie dish when it was contaminated by mold. This special mold exuded a penicillin-like substance which killed bacteria. The world of antibiotics was discovered, although implementation of his discovery took an additional ten years. Hundreds of millions of people have benefited, even though we physicians have tended to overuse antibiotics to our detriment.

In 1948, George de Mestral, an amateur Swiss mountaineer, observed the tendency of plant burrs to cling to his clothing and his dog's fur as they went for a walk. Subjecting the burrs to microscopic investigation, he saw the hooks in the plant substance which enabled the burrs to adhere to other surfaces; from this observation came the concept of Velcro, a universally applied fastening agent.

Copernicus explained his theory of heliocentrism (wherein the earth revolves around the sun, not the reverse) in 1543 C.E. Yet, in 1633 C.E., Galileo Galilei advanced the theory with his telescopic observations, only to be forced to recant his support of Copernicus's theory by the church authorities of the day. Even now, in a 1999 Gallup Poll, eighteen percent of Americans said they believed the sun revolves around the earth.

All of these pathfinders developed real-time profound insights when they paid attention to apparent anomalies. In the cases of Kekulé and Tesla, it appeared to be a matter of paying attention to creative and life-changing concepts experienced from some mysterious source deep within the minds of these exceptional observers. Old paradigms die hard and often change at a glacial pace against great resistance as humanity lurches forward, observation by observation.

Physicians and patients alike need to pay attention and be the best observers possible. In many instances, our educational system teaches us to learn rote facts, rather than learning how to think and meticulously observe all phenomena inside and outside the box in an open-minded fashion. Conventional science is revered and yet is forever changing. The certain truth of yesterday fades into the unresolved issues of today and mystery still holds much to be explored. It is important to pay attention to anomalous experiences rather than ignoring and discarding them.

I trust these stories from my journal will stimulate you to think for yourself, make your own observations, and find what works. I further trust that they will enhance your self-healing capacity and explore the margins of reality while honoring your own narrative and inviting an expanding future into your fund of knowledge for healing.

Robert A. Anderson

Citations

1. Iseri LT et al. Magnesium therapy of cardiac arrhythmias in critical-care medicine. *Magnesium* 1989; 8:299

2. McLean RM. Magnesium and its therapeutic uses: a review. *Am J Med* 1994; 96:63

3. Teo KK, Yusuf S. Role of magnesium in reducing mortality in acute myocardial infarction. A review of the evidence. *Drugs* 1993; 46:347

4. Gaby, AR. *Nutritional Medicine.* Concord, NH, Fritz Perlberg. 2011.

5. Al-Gurairi FT et al. Oral zinc sulphate in the treatment of recalcitrant viral warts: randomized placebo-controlled clinical trial. *Br J Dermatol* 2002; 146:423

6. Ellinger S, Stehle P. Efficacy of vitamin supplementation in situations with wound healing disorders: results from clinical intervention studies. *Curr Opin Clin Nutr Metab Care* 2009; 12:588

7. Moore OA. Systematic review of the use of honey as a wound dressing. *BMC Complement Altern Med* 2001; 1:2.

8. van Anholt RD et al. Specific nutritional support accelerates pressure sore healing and reduces wound care intensity in non-malnourished patients. *Nutrition* 2010; 26:867.

9. Dawson-Hughes B et al. A controlled trial of the effect of calcium supplementation on bone density in postmenopausal women. *N Engl J Med* 1990; 323:878

10. Finnerty EF. Topical zinc in the treatment of herpes simplex. *Cutis* 1986; 37:130

11. Cemek M et al. Oxidant and antioxidant levels in children with acute otitis media and tonsillitis: a comparative study. *Int J Pediatr Otorhinolaryngol* 2005; 69:823

12. Schleicher RL et al. Serum vitamin C and the prevalence of vitamin C deficiency in the United States: 2003-2004 National Health and Nutrition Examination Survey (NHANES). *Am J Clin Nutr* 2009; 90:1252.

13. Burns JJ et al. Ascorbic acid synthesis in normal and drug-treated rats, studied with L-ascorbic-1-C14 acid. *J Biol Chem* 1954 ; 207:679

14. Coca AF. *The Pulse Test*. New York, Lyle Stuart. 1956.

15. Ettelson LN et al. The value of the Coca pulse acceleration method in food allergy. *J Allergy* 1961; 32:514

16. Anderson RA. *Wellness Medicine*, New Canaan, CT, Keats. 1987.

17. Dickey LD (ed). *Clinical Ecology*. Springfield, IL, C. C. Thomas. 1976.

18. Rapp, DJ. *Is this Your Child?* New York, Harper Collins-William Morrow. 1991.

19. Pizzorno J. *Total Wellness*. Rocklin, CA, Prima. 1996.

20. Randolph TG. Ecologic orientation in medicine: comprehensive environmental control in diagnosis and therapy. *Ann Allergy* 1965; 23:7

21. Glass TA et al. Population based study of social and productive activities as predictors of survival among elderly Americans. *BMJ* 1999; 319:478

22. Lieberman J. *Take Off Your Glasses and See*. NewYork, Three Rivers Press. 1995.

23. Ivker RS, Anderson RA, Triveri L, Jr. *The Complete Self-Care Guide to Holistic Medicine*. New York, Tarcher-Putnam. 1999.

24. Hu FB et al. Diet, lifestyle and the risk of type 2 diabetes mellitus in women. *N Engl J Med* 2001; 11:790

25. Pennebaker JW. The effects of traumatic disclosure on physical and mental health: the values of writing and talking about upsetting events. *Int J Emerg Ment Health*. 1999 Winter; 1:9-18.

26. Smyth JM et al. Effects of writing about stressful experiences on symptom reduction in patients with asthma or rheumatoid arthritis: a randomized trial. *JAMA* 1999; 281:1304

27. Stauffer ER. *Unconditional Love and Forgiveness*. Whittier, CA. Triangle, 1987.

28. Goulding MM and Goulding RL. *Changing Lives Through Redecision Therapy*. NewYork, Brunner/Mazell, 1979.

29. Huggins, HA. *It's All in Your Head*. Honesdale, PA, Paragon Press. 1993.

30. Anderson JW et al. *Am J Clin Nutr* 1998 ;68(6 Suppl):1347S.

31. Pritikin N. *The Pritikin Program for Diet and Exercise.* New York, Grosset and Dunlap. 1979.

32. Rosenman RH, Friedman M. *Type A Behavior and Your Heart.* New York, Fawcett Crest, 1974.

33. Buckwalter JA. Decreasing Mobility in the Elderly. *Physician Sportsmed* 1997; 25:127

34. Benson H. *The Relaxation Response.* New York, Avon. 1975.

35. LeShan L. *How to Meditate.* New York, Little Brown. 1999.

36. Anderson RA. *Clinician's Guide to Holistic Medicine.* New York, McGraw-Hill. 2001.

37. Yue G, Cole KJ. Strength increases from the motor program: comparison of training with maximal voluntary and imagined muscle contractions. *J Neurophysiol* 1992; 67:1114

38. Zachariae R et al. Effect of psychological intervention in the form of relaxation and guided imagery on cellular immune function in normal healthy subjects. An overview. *Psychother Psychosom* 1990; 54:32

39. Assagioli RA. *The Act of Will.* New York, Viking. 1973.

40. O'Regan, B, Hirschberg C. *Spontaneous Remission.* Sausalito, CA, Institute of Noetic Sciences. 1993.

41. Dowling SJ. Lourdes cures and their medical assessment. *J R Soc Med* 1984; 77:634

42. Riordan HD et al. A pilot clinical study of continuous intravenous ascorbate in terminal cancer patients. *P R Health Sci J* 2005; 24:269

43. Cathcart RF. Vitamin C: the nontoxic, non-rate-limited, antioxidant free radical scavenger. *Med Hypotheses* 1985; 18:61

44. Chen Q et al. Pharmacologic ascorbic acid concentrations selectively kill cancer cells: action as a pro-drug to deliver hydrogen peroxide to tissues. *Proc Natl Acad Sci U S A* 2005; 102:13604

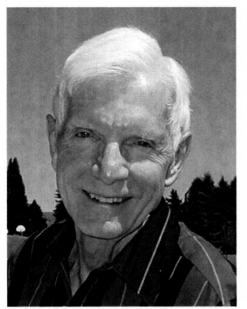

Robert Anderson, MD graduated with honors from medical school in 1957 and practiced family medicine for 40 years in Edmonds, Washington. He was the Founding Chief of Staff at Stevens Memorial Hospital in Edmonds, the founding president of the American Board of Integrative Holistic Medicine in 1996, and Adjunct Instructor in Family Medicine at Bastyr University in Kenmore, Washington, since 1992. He was elected as a charter fellow of the American Academy of Family Physicians, a diplomate of the American Board of Family Practice (1973-1991), and Clinical Assistant Professor of Family Medicine at the University of Washington (1976-89) .

He has conducted thousands of classes, workshops and seminars in stress management and integrative holistic medicine in North America, Central America, Europe and New Zealand. His published books include *Clinician's Guide to Holistic Medicine* (2001), *Wellness Medicine* (1987), and *Stress Power* (1978).

Bob and his wife Joann raised three children and have two grandchildren. He maintains an avid interest in hiking, skiing, and political action.

Teeth - Pg 11
rattling hip 19
R Arthritis 37
insomnia 41 no choc milk...
weight loss 43
50 - old age 48
eyes 52
Diabetes 55
Volunteering for life 60
diarrhea 63
hysteria 66
grieving forgiveness & heart disease 69

CPSIA information can be obtained at www.ICGtesting.com
Printed in the USA
BVOW012022191011

273440BV00001BA/2/P

9 780983 742210